P9-CFP-644

The 7-Day Flat-Belly
Tea Cleanse

The Revolutionary New Plan to
Melt Up to 10 Pounds
in Just One Week!

KELLY CHOI
and the Editors of
EAT THIS, NOT THAT!®

No book can replace the diagnostic expertise and medical advice of a trusted physician. Please be certain to consult with your doctor before making any decisions that affect your health, particularly if you suffer from any medical condition or have any symptom that may require treatment.

Mention of specific companies, organizations, or authorities in this book does not imply endorsement by the author or publisher, nor does mention of specific companies, organizations, or authorities imply that they endorse this book, its author, or the publisher.

Copyright © 2015 by David Zinczenko

All rights reserved.

Published in the United States by Galvanized Books, a division of Galvanized Brands, LLC, New York

Galvanized Books is a trademark of Galvanized Brands, LLC

ISBN 978-1-940358-03-1

Design by Mike Smith

Kelly Choi and tea photographs by Terry Doyle
Styling by Argy Koutsothanasis
Hair and makeup by Daniella @ WorkGroup

GALVANIZED

The 7-Day Flat-Belly Tea Cleanse

TABLE OF CONTENTS

INTRODUCTION

Tea saved my mother's life. It changed my life. And I believe it will change yours.

Shortly after I was born, my mother developed diabetes. It runs in our family; I lost an uncle to the disease, and I have other relatives who struggle with it.

My parents met in South Korea when they worked together at a hospital—my mother as a nurse, my father as a pharmacist. When I turned 3 we immigrated to America, but language barriers prevented them from pursuing their former careers, so they did what so many educated Koreans have done: They opened a grocery store.

Owning a convenience store is not a good career for a diabetic; everywhere you look, you're surrounded by muffins, doughnuts, candy bars. Growing up, I enjoyed all the baked goods I could eat, times 10.

Then, five years ago, my father passed away from complications from a stroke. Shortly afterward, my mother had a terrible fall. Her diabetes was raging out of control.

THE 7-DAY FLAT-BELLY TEA CLEANSE

I remember the day I sat with her, after doctors had told her the limitations of Western medicine when it came to diabetes. I asked her about her time as a nurse in Korea, and what she knew of Eastern medicine. And the same word kept coming up time and again:

Tea.

It had been a common drink in our house when I was young, but over time we moved away from this life-saving drink toward commercial soft drinks. During a short stint back in Korea, I had rediscovered tea for myself. Now, with my mother's life at stake, I knew I had to act.

I threw myself into the research, using my parents' medical background and my own skills as a journalist and dedicated foodie. And what I discovered—and what's outlined here in *The 7-Day Flat-Belly Tea Cleanse*—is a mountain of stunning evidence that tea can not only help strip away unwanted pounds and bring blood sugar under control but can ward off most of the worst diseases of our time, while helping to strip away stress and give us back control of our lives.

I tried this cleanse myself, and within 48 hours my waist was measurably smaller, and I felt lighter, more alert, and yet more calm. I shared it with my mother, and her 7-day journey brought her blood sugar under control, and her weight down by a shocking 9 pounds.

And then she and I shared it with our friends, and the results were the same across the board. In just 48 to 72 hours, our friends reported noticeable changes in their body shapes, as though the tea were flattening their bellies from the inside. Seven days was all it took to strip off 6, 8, 10 pounds.

Now, I want to share this remarkable program with you. Complete with simple, easy and delicious recipes, and an easy-to-follow cleanse regimen, *The 7-Day Flat-Belly Tea Cleanse* has changed my life, and the lives of the people I love.

And it's going to change yours as well.

INTRODUCTION

SIP AWAY STRESS, SIP AWAY POUNDS

Imagine for a moment that you're walking down the beach. The sand is moist and cool below your feet. Seagulls caw overhead, and the waves shush your nerves and soothe your troubles as they caress the beach and slowly slink back. All is calm.

Up ahead, half buried in the sand, you see an antique container of some sort, washed up on the shore after centuries of tossing around in the ocean. A bowl? A lantern? No, it's an ornate teakettle, lost in the sinking of a great Spanish galleon. You lift it up, rub the side, and suddenly—poof! A genie appears. And he makes you an offer: He's going to give you a magic potion that can strip pounds from your body, improve your health, make you more attractive to your mate, and keep you lean for life.

What is this potion?

Tea.

I know what you're thinking: Mr. Genie, don't you mean I should head down to the supplement store and buy some of that super-expensive stuff that tastes like cocoa powder mixed with Pepto-Bismol? Surely, good old tea doesn't have magical weight-loss powers, does it?

In fact, that's exactly what we're talking about here. Tea: the stuff of curled pinkie fingers and crumpets and aunties with too many cats. The stuff they threw off the boat in Boston to protest British taxation. (Maybe that's where America's obesity problem began?) More and more research has shown that different types of tea possess different micronutrients that do everything from revving your metabolism to blocking the formation of new fat cells to actually working on your body at a genetic level, reversing your inherited tendency to gain weight and making it easy—effortless, in fact—to drop pounds quickly.

Literally hundreds of studies have been carried out to document the health benefits of catechins, the group of antioxidants concentrated in the leaves of tea plants. Among the most startling studies was one published by the American Medical Association. The study followed more than 40,000 Japanese adults for a decade, and at the 7-year follow-up, those who had been drinking five or more cups of tea per day during the initial study were 26 percent less likely to die of any cause compared with those who averaged less than a cup.

Looking for more immediate results? Another Japanese study broke participants into two groups, only one of which was put on a tea-rich diet. At the end of 12 weeks, the tea group had achieved significantly smaller body weights and waistlines than those in the control group. Why? Because researchers believe that catechins, the nutrients that give tea its nutritional punch, are effective at boosting metabolism.

IN A 10-YEAR JAPANESE STUDY, THOSE WHO DRANK THE MOST GREEN TEA WERE LESS LIKELY TO DIE OF ANY CAUSE THROUGHOUT THE COURSE OF THE STUDY.

This book is a complete 7-day plan for jump-starting your natural fat burners while tapping the incredible health-boosting powers of tea. In addition, I'll provide you with a healthy, sensible eating plan that reinforces the magical powers of your favorite teas and strips away pounds, abracadabra.

You may have seen or even tried other "cleanses" before, but the Tea Cleanse is different. You'll get to eat food—which means you'll keep your metabolism revving—plus delicious smoothies that have all of the nutrients and fiber so often missing from more common juice cleanses. Because of that, you won't have to deal with the hunger, fatigue and irritability so common among those who try traditional cleanses—in part because juice cleanses can be so high in sugar. No hunger, no deprivation, just rapid, sustainable weight loss. If it all sounds too good to be true, then I ask you to give me just 3 days. I have seen dramatic results in just 72 hours from men and women just like you who have followed this delicious plan—without the need for exercise or calorie restriction, without giving up their favorite foods, and without ever feeling hungry or deprived. You'll be shocked to discover the needle on the scale start to move and the tightness at your waist start to ease in the course of just one long weekend.

In fact, you'll be shocked to discover just how many benefits you'll reap from this simple, delicious and naturally healthy program.

___

YOU'LL LOSE BODY FAT—EVEN AS YOU ENJOY YOUR FAVORITE FOODS.

Japanese researchers found that levels of antioxidants called polymerized polyphenols, found in certain teas, inhibit the body's ability to absorb fat by as much as 20 percent. (It's like a get-out-of-jail-free card!) When Taiwanese researchers studied more than 1,100 people over a 10-year period, they determined that those who drank black, green or oolong tea had nearly 20 percent less body fat than those who drank none.

YOU'LL LOWER YOUR BLOOD PRESSURE.

According to a study in the *Archives of Internal Medicine*, people who consumed 120 milliliters of tea every day for at least a year had 46 percent lower risk of developing hypertension than those who consumed less.

YOU'LL STRENGTHEN YOUR BONES.

Chinese scientists exposed bone cells to catechins, the nutrients found in certain teas. The nutrients actually helped the bones to grow, and slowed the breakdown of bone cells. One of the catechins boosted bone growth by 79 percent. And a 2105 study at Osaka University in Japan found that theaflavin-3 (TF-3), an antioxidant in tea, inhibits the function of an enzyme called DNA methyltransferase, which destroys bone tissue as we age. The study, published in the U.S. journal *Nature Medicine*, found that when mice suffering from osteoporosis were given TF-3, they showed recovering levels of bone volume, similar to those of healthy mice. Researchers said that drinking about 20 cups of tea a day would show results in as little as three days.

YOU'LL MAKE YOUR IMMUNE SYSTEM STRONGER.

In a study published in the *Proceedings of the National Academy of Sciences*, those who drank 20 ounces of black tea daily secreted 5 times more interferon, a key element of your body's infection-protection arsenal.

YOU'LL SLOW THE AGING PROCESS.

According to a Case Western Reserve University study, an extract of white tea leaves may help fight wrinkles and keep your skin looking young. "Chemicals in the tea appear to protect your skin from sun-induced stress, which can cause the cells to break down prematurely," says Elma Baron, M.D., the study author.

YOU'LL REDUCE STRESS AND SLEEP BETTER.

You probably already know that chamomile tea can help induce sleep. (There's even a brand called Sleepytime.) But science is showing that teas actually work on a hormonal level to lower our agita and bring peace and slumber. Studies have found that rooibos tea contains compounds that can actually reduce levels of stress hormones in our bodies, bringing on sleep—and reducing the body's ability to store fat!

YOU'LL LOWER YOUR RISK OF CANCER AND OTHER THREATS TO YOUR HEALTH AND HAPPINESS.

A recent study at Penn State found that EGCG, one of the active ingredients in green tea, triggers a virtuous cycle that kills off oral cancer cells. "EGCG does something to damage the mitochondria" of cancer cells, says Joshua Lambert, associate professor of food science at Penn State's Center for Plant and Mushroom Foods for Health. Yet at the same time, it also boosts the protective capabilities of the normal cells surrounding the cancer cells.

Ready to give it a try? Here's how to start drinking up—and start slimming down!

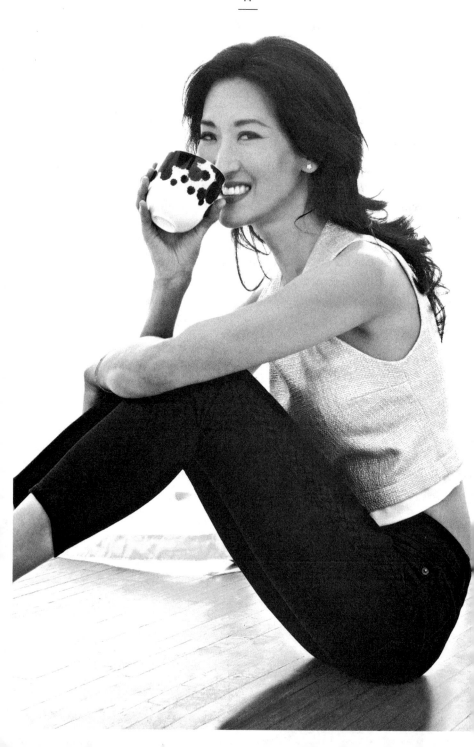

Sip Off the Pounds

Six simple steps before you begin

Before you begin *The 7-Day Flat-Belly Tea Cleanse*, take a moment to think about your past drinking habits. No, not that time in college when you got arrested for streaking through the quad at 1 a.m. I mean the stuff you drink every

SIP OFF THE POUNDS

day: sodas, sweet teas, energy drinks, lattes, juices and the like.

The average American now drinks about a gallon of soda a week. Add to that our odd new habits of swapping tap water for bottled "vitamin" water (+120 calories) and giving up plain iced coffee for Mocha Frappucinos (+520 calories) and you can see how quickly the calories add up—and that's before chugging an "energy drink" that tastes exactly like what would happen if a crazed pastry chef hijacked a truckload of Smarties and drove it into a battery acid factory (another 280 calories). Those three drinks alone give you 920 additional calories—almost half a day's worth!

In fact, liquid calories now make up a whopping 21 percent of our daily calorie intake—more than 400 calories every single day, more than twice as much as we drank 30 years ago. To give you a perspective on those numbers, imagine taking two slices of Pizza Hut Thin 'N Crispy Pepperoni Pizza, tossing them in a blender and hitting "puree," then drinking the whole thing down. That's 420 calories. Now imagine that the typical American has been doing this every single day for years.

Wow. Disgusting, right?

Yes, but behind those slightly sickening statistics comes some great news. Because if you want to strip away pounds, shrink your belly, and begin to sculpt a leaner, fitter body—while also boosting your health, calming your mind and fighting back against some of the most significant diseases of our time—just changing what you drink could be all you need.

One study at Johns Hopkins University found that people who cut liquid calories from their diets lose more weight—and keep it off longer—than people who cut food calories. Simply cutting out liquid calories—by switching your usual drink to tea—could save you nearly 42 pounds this year alone! (Sorta makes that genie look real, doesn't it?)

So to start using the Tea Cleanse, you first have to rid yourself of the liquid toxins your body has been piling up. Here's how to do it:

STEP 1

SWEAR OFF THE SODA AND BOTTLED TEAS

ANNUAL WEIGHT LOSS: 12 POUNDS

According to the National Institutes of Health, the third largest source of food calories in the American diet isn't a food at all. It's soda. We get more calories from soda every day than we do meat, dairy or anything other than baked goods. How can that be possible? Because of all the sugar. Mountain Dew, for example, not only delivers 52 grams of sugar per 12-ounce can, but gives you a delicious side helping of bromated vegetable oil, a component of rocket fuel. And I don't mean metaphorical rocket fuel—I mean the stuff they actually put in the engines to keep the gears from exploding.

STEP 2

DON'T DRINK JUICE DRINKS

ANNUAL WEIGHT LOSS: 19 POUNDS

If the FDA ever forces drink manufacturers to start properly labeling their products, SunnyD would have to be called Obesi-D. (Some versions of the brand have up to 180 calories and 40 grams of sugar per serving.) Most of these "juice" drinks are really just water and high-fructose corn syrup. If you drink just one of these a day, cut it out— you'll lose 19 pounds this year!

STEP 3

TRADE COFFEE DRINKS FOR TEA

ANNUAL WEIGHT LOSS: 25 POUNDS

Researchers studied the coffee habits of New Yorkers and discovered that two-thirds of Starbucks customers opted for blended coffee drinks over regular brewed coffee or tea. The average caloric impact of the blended drinks was 239 calories. Switch to tea just once a day and you'd lose 25 pounds this year! (Actually, you may lose more, as coffee has been linked to belly fat storage. A research team in Washington found that five or more cups of Joe a day doubled visceral fat.)

STEP 4

USE TEA TO "FLAVOR" YOUR WATER

ANNUAL WEIGHT LOSS: 13½ POUNDS

In one of the greatest feats of marketing ever, Vitaminwater produces products that sound a lot like health drinks but are nothing more than straight-up sugar. Its Power-C Dragonfruit flavored water has 120 calories and 31 grams of sugar—that's the equivalent of drinking 13 Jolly Ranchers. You would lose more than a pound a month just by making this one swap each day.

STEP 5

CHOOSE TEA OVER JUICE

ANNUAL WEIGHT LOSS: 14½ POUNDS

What could be healthier than this: Langers Pomegranate Blueberry Plus. It's 100 percent juice, says so right on the label. But the "Plus" is juice concentrate, which is so sweet that Langers packs 30 grams of sugar in each 8 ounce glass: that's the sugar equivalent of two—two!—Snicker's Ice Cream Bars.

STEP 6

MAKE YOUR OWN ICED TEA

ANNUAL WEIGHT LOSS: 13½ POUNDS

If you're a Snapple fan, you probably saw "Tea Cleanse" and thought, Great! But bottled teas aren't necessarily the answer. First, once a tea is made and sits on a supermarket shelf for, oh, an entire NFL season, the nutrients have spent enough time exposed to light and air that they begin to break down. Plus, who knows what else has worked its way into that bottle? Snapple's All Natural Green Tea packs 120 calories and 30 grams of sugar, while Ssips Green Tea with Honey & Ginseng is sweetened not so much with honey but with high-fructose corn syrup.

DON'T HIT THE BOTTLE

A few years back, the authors of Eat This, Not That! commissioned ChromaDex laboratories to analyze 14 different bottled green teas for their levels of disease-fighting catechins. While Honest Tea Honey Green Tea topped the charts with an impressive 215 milligrams of total catechins, some products weren't even in the game. For instance, Republic of Tea Pomegranate Green Tea had only 8 milligrams, and Ito En Teas' Tea Lemongrass Green had just 28 milligrams, despite implying on its label that the product is packed with antioxidants.

Why the discrepancy? The fact is, store-bought teas typically lose 20 percent of EGCG/catechin content during the bottling process, which is why brewing your own is so critical. If you really want bottled tea then shoot for versions with an acid like lemon juice or citric acid, which help stabilize EGCG levels. Recent studies show that the more acidic the environment, the more stable the tea's nutrients. But even in a highly acidic drink, more than half of the nutrients are gone within 3 months.

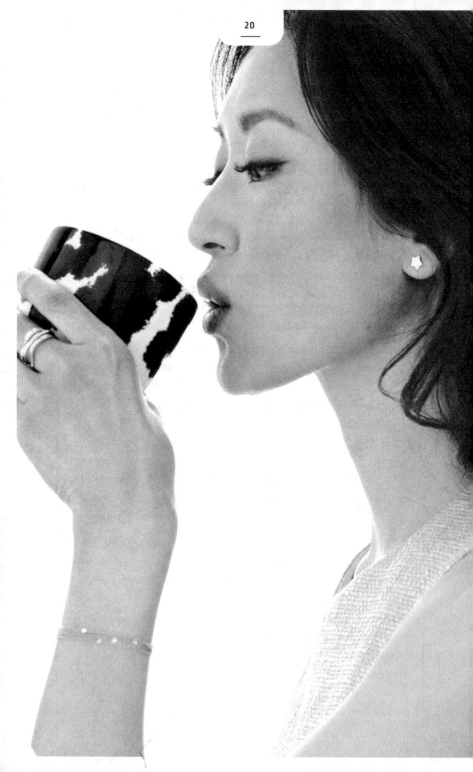

The Principles of the Tea Cleanse

How to use this plan to strip away up to 14 pounds in just 7 days!

I believe in *The 7-Day Flat-Belly Tea Cleanse* because I've seen the power of tea, and I've experienced it for myself. Tea saved my mother's life, and has changed the lives of so many people I know.

THE PRINCIPLES OF THE TEA CLEANSE

Tea has not only given me control over my body, my health, and my weight, but it has also given me something far more valuable: control over my mind, my stress, and my time.

It was during a short time in Seoul, South Korea, while I was pursuing a media career, that my love affair with tea truly began. In Korea, tea is as common as bottled water in America. Everywhere you look, vending machines are selling not cans of Coke but 60-cent cups of hot tea. And so, wanting to fit in, I too joined the tea culture.

And that's when everything changed. Tea will literally squelch your appetite and make staying slim utterly effortless. When you drink tea, you do more than nourish yourself. You join an international community of people around the world who are engaging in the very same rituals as you. Throughout Asia, tea is practically a national drink. In places like Morocco, you'll never enter a home without being offered tea—it's considered rude! From England to India, people plan their travel and work schedules around tea.

And tea is both a private and a social event. Nobody thinks of getting together for a soda; drinking alone isn't a very good sign; and coffee is a great drink, but one that comes with its own jittery side effects. Tea stands alone as the ritual you can enjoy alone before bedtime, or with a close girlfriend catching up on the latest gossip.

And that's why only tea makes sense as the basis of a cleanse that you can revisit over and over again. You don't have to order it from a fancy delivery service, spend oodles of your hard-earned dough on proprietary concoctions, or become a monk who can't join in social events because there's none of your magic elixir on hand. If you have a few dimes and access to hot water, you've got it made.

I've already shared with you the power of this amazing brew. Now I want to share with you the principles of the Tea Cleanse, so you can begin experiencing its magic immediately.

The 7-Day Flat-Belly Tea Cleanse
Cheat Sheet

▬ HOT TEAS

You'll enjoy one nourishing cup of tea, five times a day, during the cleanse. Each is carefully selected to provide your body with the maximum benefits it needs at the very time that it needs it.

- One metabolism-boosting tea to rev up your fat burners
- One flat-belly tea to fight inflammation and reduce bloating
- Two fat-blocking teas (one before dinner and one before your midday Tea Cleanse Smoothie) to shrink your fat cells, prevent weight gain, and reduce hunger
- One stress-busting tea to improve focus and ensure better sleep

▬ MEALS

There is no breakfast on this plan. Instead, you'll replace breakfast with a metabolism-boosting tea to force your body to burn stored fat for energy. For lunch, you'll enjoy a filling and delicious Tea Cleanse Smoothie. And for dinner, you'll have a complete, nourishing and satisfying meal. As a result, you'll strip 800-1,700 calories out of each and every day while still feeling full and energized.

TEA CLEANSE SMOOTHIES

Every day, you're going to look forward to enjoying a cool, creamy and delicious tea smoothie. These recipes will keep you full while ensuring your body has all of the fat-melting nutrients it needs to amp up your weight loss to the max.

MORNING RITUAL

You'll begin every day not with some sort of horrible exercise routine or nose-crinkling potion, but with a gentle walk in the sunshine. All you need is 10 minutes each day to trigger the ingredients in your morning tea to start working their magic.

The 7-Day Flat-Belly Tea Cleanse
Meal Plan

7 am 1-2 cups Metabolism-Boosting tea (your choice of green, oolong, yerba mate, goji, kola nut)

7:30 am Morning ritual (10- to 30-minute walk, preferably outdoors)

10 am 1 cup Fat-Blocker Tea (your choice of white, green, black, barberry, rooibos, pu-erh)

12 pm 8-ounce Tea Cleanse Smoothie

3 pm 1 cup Flat-Belly Tea (your choice of mint, ginger, bilberry, hibiscus, fennel, lemon)

6 pm 1 cup Fat-Blocker Tea (your choice of white, green, black, barberry, rooibos, pu-erh)

7 pm Tea Cleanse Dinner

9 pm 1 cup Stress-Busting Tea (your choice of kava kava, ashwangandha, passionflower, hops, rooibos, lemon balm, valerian, chamomile with lavender)

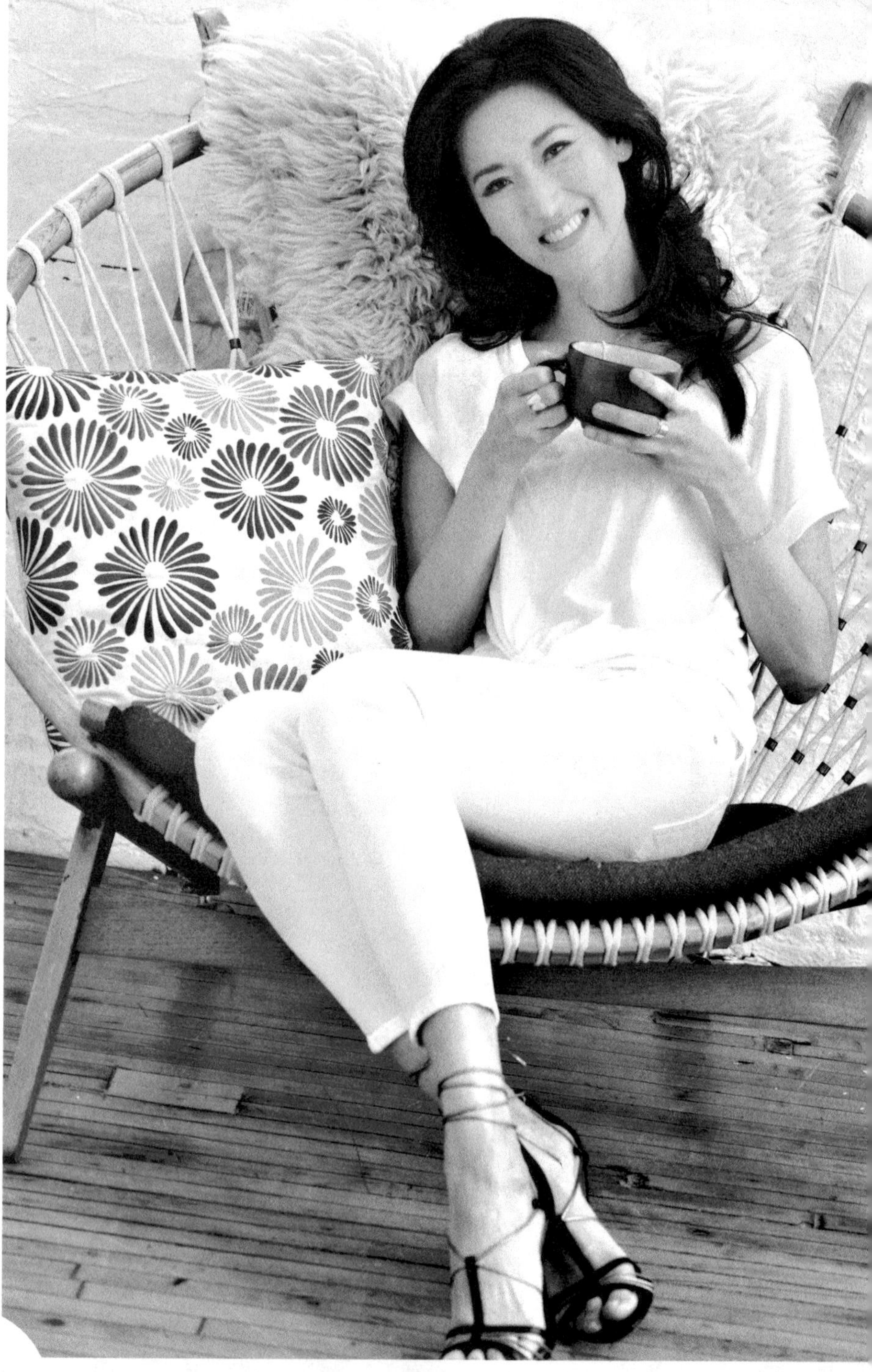

The Rules of Tea

How to brew and understand tea for maximum weight loss

If you're like most Americans, when you hear the word *tea* the first thing that comes to mind is a yellow box from Lipton, or a bottle of Snapple, or a commercial of a guy taking the Nestea plunge.

THE RULES OF TEA

You probably know that green tea is good for you, that a hot tea with honey soothes the throat, and that chai is a flavoring you get at Starbucks.

And that's about it.

But when it comes to our attitude toward tea, we're pretty much alone in the world. From the cold shores of the British Isles to the steamy jungles of Southeast Asia, tea is a critical daily component of many cultures, as ritualized and debated there as craft brews and the NFL draft are here. In many regions, tea leaves are considered as nuanced and diverse as wine grapes. In Japan, an entire formal ceremony is built around the preparation of matcha, a form of green tea; in some parts of the former British empire, folks still break at 4 p.m. or so for tea time each day. And like many other cultural rituals, the rituals that formed around tea have a basis in physical and spiritual health. In the coming pages, you'll read more about how to prepare tea and use it as your secret weight-loss weapon.

And the good news is that you don't need to have manservants, a geisha, a special tea hut, or even a pair of white gloves to enjoy the maximum flavor and health benefits of tea. But you should keep a few rules in mind if you want to extract all the weight-loss muscle that teas have to offer.

The Traditional Tea Types

Much like human beings, teas come in all sorts of colors and extractions, from all sorts of regions and national backgrounds, and with all sorts of flavors and temperaments. And like humans, teas all have unique and wonderful attributes. What you want to shoot for, both as part of your Tea Cleanse and for general health benefits now and in the future, is to seek out as much diversity as possible. Just as eating a wide variety of fruits and vegetables will help ensure you have a full range of vitamins and minerals, so too will sipping an array of teas guarantee a maximum intake of the belly-flattening, stress-busting, health-boosting micronutrients found in these delicious brews.

The Tea Cleanse plan organizes the teas below by their unique powers—to boost metabolism, reduce fat storage, quash hunger and reduce stress—and puts each to work at different times during the day. But as you embrace tea as part of a healthy lifestyle, you'll no doubt want to keep your palate intrigued by seeking out subcategories and special varieties. Here are the main types you need to know:

GREEN TEA

ORIGINS: China, Japan, Southeast Asia
ALSO KNOWN AS: Jasmine (a blend of green tea infused with jasmine flowers), Pinhead Gunpowder, sencha, Chinese tea, Japanese tea, matcha, Dragon Well, Pu-erh

THE RULES OF TEA

CAFFEINE CONTENT: 15–20mg per cup

CRUCIAL FACTS: People who consume at least 120ml of green tea—that's about half a cup—each day for at least a year have a 46 percent lower risk of developing hypertension than those who consume less, according to a study in the *Archives of Internal Medicine.*

WHITE TEA

ORIGINS: China

ALSO KNOWN AS: Silver needle, white peony, long life eyebrow

CAFFEINE CONTENT: 45–60mg per cup

CRUCIAL FACTS: A study from Case Western Reserve University found that chemicals in white tea appear to protect skin from sun-induced stress, preventing premature aging.

BLACK TEA

ORIGINS: India, Sri Lanka, Argentina, China

ALSO KNOWN AS: English breakfast, Irish breakfast, Assam, Ceylon, Darjeeling, Earl Grey (a blend of black teas scented with bergamot oil), chai (black tea spiked with spices—more on this below)

CAFFEINE CONTENT: 40–120mg per cup

CRUCIAL FACTS: Drinking 20 ounces of black tea daily causes the body to secrete five times as much interferon, a key element of your body's infection-protection arsenal.

OOLONG TEA

ORIGINS: China, Taiwan

ALSO KNOWN AS: Oolong has no other names. Who would pass up the chance to say "oolong"?

CAFFEINE CONTENT: 35–45mg per cup

CRUCIAL FACTS: Traditionalists believe that oolong tea leaves should be "washed," which basically means throwing out your first cup. Pour hot water over the leaves, let them infuse for 10 seconds, then discard the water. (This treatment supposedly "wakes up" the flavor.) Now pour in more hot water and steep for up to 4 minutes.

RED TEA

ORIGINS: South Africa

ALSO KNOWN AS: Rooibos, bush tea

CAFFEINE CONTENT: Zero

CRUCIAL FACTS: Rooibos leaves are very small, so use a fine filter and don't steep for more than a couple of minutes; the small leaves create a very intense, sweet flavor.

MATE

ORIGINS: South America

ALSO KNOWN AS: Yerba mate

CAFFEINE CONTENT: Zero. Mate contains a caffeine-like substance called mateine, which has a stimulant effect without the jitteriness of caffeine.

CRUCIAL FACTS: While more research needs to be done, mateine's effects on metabolism are so highly valued that mate is listed as an ingredient in many diet pills. To get the benefits of mate without the dangerous side effects of pills, use a tea sack filled with 1 heaping teaspoon of mate for every 12 ounces of water, and steep for 1 to 4 minutes.

HERBAL TEAS

ORIGINS: various

ALSO KNOWN AS: Tisane, chamomile, hibiscus, anise, peppermint, lemon balm, burdock, cinnamon, citrus, ginger, valerian, lavender, hops, passionflower, ashwagandha, kava kava

CAFFEINE CONTENT: Zero

CRUCIAL FACTS: "Herbal tea" basically refers to any kind of herb, flower, spice, or other plant material soaked in hot water—they aren't technically teas at all. A proper tea comes from a variation of the tea plant (*Camellia sinensis*). However, since many specific herbal teas have stress-relieving properties, which can help improve general health and set the table for weight loss, they will become a regular part of your evening ritual.

No-Trouble Brewing

If you can boil water, you can make tea. But here's the irony: If you can boil water, you can also ruin a good cup of tea, at least according to aficionados and health experts. By tweaking your tea ever so slightly, you can ensure you're getting maximum flavor and maximum health benefits. Here's how:

Don't hold the bag. Consider investing in loose tea leaves. While tea bags are the cheapest, fastest, and most convenient ways to get your tea fix, a report by ConsumerLab.com, an independent site that tests health products, found that green tea brewed from loose tea leaves yielded the highest levels of catechins, an antioxidant found in plants that gives tea much of its weight-loss benefits. (You'll read more about catechins in the coming chapters.) The report compared a single teaspoonful of Teavana's Gyokuro green tea with single bags of green tea sold by Lipton and Bigelow. Researchers found that the loose green tea yielded about 250mg of catechins, while the tea bags yielded slightly less. But loose tea is more expensive: The report calculated that to obtain 200mg of epigallocatechin gallate, or EGCG—a particularly potent form of catechin that's been shown to "turn off" the genes that trigger obesity, diabetes, and the storage of belly fat—you'd spend between 27 and 60 cents using tea bags versus $2.18 using loose tea leaves. In addition, folic acid, a B vitamin found in tea that also helps the body resist weight gain and diabetes, is found in high quantities in both loose and bagged teas. But a study in the *Journal of the American Dietetic Association* found that tea bags themselves can inhibit the transfer of folic acid.

Get your matcha on. Matcha is a form of green tea that uses the entire leaf in powdered form, rather than flakes of leaves. Matcha is a ceremonial tea that is gaining in popularity and

THE RULES OF TEA

becoming more widely available. Because the powdered tea dissolves directly into the water (and you can brew it hot or cold), some believe that a greater percentage of the nutrients in matcha become available to your body than with standard green teas. Be aware that there are different grades of matcha; while China is now producing this product to varying degrees of success, the best matcha comes from Japan, and will be a bright green. Knockoffs may be brownish and bitter.

Hit the right temperature. When the teakettle blows, take the water off of the heat and let it rest for about 30 seconds, says Linda Smith, owner and master tea blender at Divinitea.com. "Boiling water scorches tea, which gives it a tart, tannic taste," she explains. And, much like overcooking vegetables, intensely boiling water may damage some of the delicate nutrients you're looking to extract. Give the water time to come down from its 212 degree boiling point to about 185 degrees (even a little less for delicate green tea) before you add it to your tea leaves.

Know your brew times. A study in the *Journal of Agricultural Food Chemistry* looked at six popular brands of tea and demonstrated that with each type of tea, there is a careful balance between getting the maximum level of nutrients, and turning the tea bitter. "The difference between a really good cup and not is to remember to take the leaves out," says Smith. "If you leave them in too long, the cup becomes too strong."

Black and mate teas need about 3 to 5 minutes to steep to achieve maximum antioxidant capacity.

Green and oolong teas need 2 to 3 minutes of steeping time.

White teas are also ready in 2 to 3 minutes, but because of their delicate flavor, you may want to steep up to 5 minutes to get a robustness more in line with the American palate.

Rooibos tea, because it releases its flavor so quickly, can be ready in 2 minutes or less. Experiment with time to get the right flavor for you.

Use a little lemon to maximize your benefits.

When you sip tea, a significant percentage of the polyphenol antioxidants break down before they reach your bloodstream. But researchers at Purdue University discovered that adding lemon juice to the equation helped preserve the polyphenols.

Ditch the dairy. A study in the *European Heart Journal*

found that while tea can improve blood flow and blood-vessel dilation (and thereby lower your blood pressure), adding milk to the tea counteracts these effects.

Sun Tease

When summer comes, traditionalists like to create "sun tea," a cold-brewing method that involves setting a clear pitcher of cold water on a windowsill with four to six tea bags inside and allowing the power of the sun to draw the flavor and nutrients out of the tea bags over the course of an afternoon.

Not having to light a stove or fill the kitchen with steam during a sweltering summer's day makes a lot of sense, and the mellower flavor is often preferred for unsweetened iced teas. But according to a study in *Journal of Food Processing and Preservation*, cold-water brewing is not as effective at extracting catechins (or caffeine) from tea leaves. Another study in *Food Science and Technology* found that total catechins were about 16 percent lower in cold-brewed teas than in those made with hot water. If this hot summer method still appeals, feel free, but be aware that you may be enjoying a drink that's not as impactful as your standard tea drink.

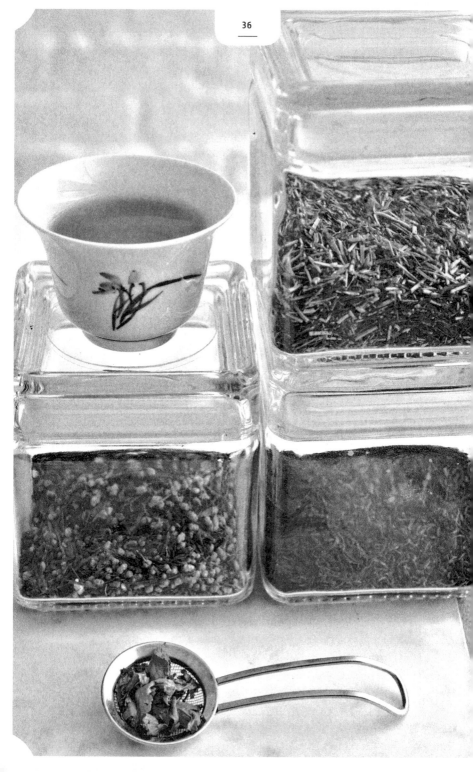

Fat-Blocking Teas

The best teas for shutting down
your fat-storage system and
telling your fat cells to flake off!

A steaming cup of tea is the
perfect drink for soothing
a sore throat, warming up on
a cold winter's night, or
binge-watching *Downton
Abbey.* But certain teas are also
perfect for doing something

else—helping you lose weight. Or, more specifically, preventing your body from being able to gain weight.

Think of your body as an always-changing, amorphous entity. In this ongoing battle, you're always getting a little bit leaner or a little bit heavier. And while intense exercise and restrictive diets will move the needle on a short-term basis, a simple cup or two of tea will nudge you in the right direction, just a little, over and over again, day after day after day. It's exactly the kind of weight loss you want—the kind that doesn't require any extraordinary effort on your part, but when you run into people you haven't seen in a while, eyebrows raise: "How did you do it?"

You may (or may not) want to share your secrets: six teas that block fat and make weight loss automatic. You only need one of the below tea types on any given day—some folks stick with the same tea day after day, while others like to purchase a variety and mix it up each day. It's all up to you and your taste buds.

THE BELLY CONDUCTOR
WHITE TEA

DRINK THIS: Twinings, The Republic of Tea, Celestial Seasonings Sleepytime

BECAUSE IT: Shuttles fat from the body

White tea is dried naturally, often in sunlight, making it the least processed and richest source of antioxidants among teas (as much as three times as many polyphenols as green tea!).

In fact, white tea works in four distinct ways to help strip fat from your body. A study published in the *Journal of Nutrition and Metabolism* showed that white tea can simultaneously boost lipolysis (the breakdown of fat) and block adipogenesis (the formation of fat cells) due to high levels of ingredients thought to be active on human fat cells. Another group of researchers found that the tea is also a rich source of a type of antioxidant that triggers the release of fat from the cells and helps speed the liver's ability to turn fat into energy. Who needs Spanx when you can just sip on this powerful brew? If there's such a thing as diet tea, this is it.

THE FAT-GENE HACKER
GREEN TEA

DRINK THIS: Lipton, Yogi

BECAUSE IT: Reverses your fat-storage genes

Green tea or its derivatives appear on your Tea Cleanse schedule every day for good reason—in fact, for a wide array of reasons. Green tea is particularly high in a type of catechin called EGCG, which can "turn off" the genetic triggers for diabetes and obesity.

If that sounds like science fiction, it's not: It's the new science of nutritional genetics, and it's changing everything we know about weight loss. A 2014 study in the journal *Advanced Nutrition* found that obese and diabetic people have different patterns of gene

FAT-BLOCKING TEAS

markers than those who are not obese or diabetic. Essentially, say the researchers, the "on" switches for their fat-storage genes have been tripped. In another review of 46 different studies on the topic of obesity and genetics, researchers writing in the *International Journal of Obesity* in 2014 reported that genetic markers for obesity—evidence that fat genes have been turned on—can be spotted at birth, and those markers can predict whether a newborn will become obese as an adult.

"What you eat, and don't eat, can influence which genes are turned on and when," says Kevin L. Schalinske, Ph.D., professor in the Department of Food Science and Human Nutrition at Iowa State University. And it can turn those genes back off. Once they're off, it becomes hard for your body to gain weight—it's simply not predisposed to pack on the pounds. Researchers have identified 11 nutrients that turn off fat genes, including those found in fruits, nuts, and eggs. But green tea is unique among foods because it is the best possible source of one of the most important fat-gene reversal switches, ECGC. It also contains folate, a second trigger food that turns off genetic switches for weight gain and insulin resistance.

EGCG also boosts levels of cholecystokinin, or CCK, a hunger-quelling hormone. In a Swedish study that looked at green tea's effect on hunger, researchers divided up participants into two groups: One group sipped water with their meals and the other group drank green tea. Not only did tea sippers report less of a desire to eat their favorite foods (even two hours after sipping the brew), they found those foods to be less satisfying. And a 2015 study from the Institute of Food Research found that the polyphenols in green tea block the "signaling molecule" called vascular endothelial growth factor, or VEGF, which in the body can trigger both heart disease and cancer.

THE FAT-HORMONE STOPPER
BLACK TEA

DRINK THIS: Bigelow, Lipton

BECAUSE IT: Reduces your body's levels of fat-storage hormones

Screaming babies. Screaming bosses. Screaming cable news anchors. Whatever your source of stress, it's important to realize that these factors aren't just making you frazzled—they're making you fat.

Stress is a major contributor to weight gain. See, our bodies simply aren't designed to handle modern life. When stress hits, the first thing that happens is that your body jacks up its production of adrenaline. Adrenaline causes fat cells all over your body to squirt their stores of fatty acids into your bloodstream to be used as energy. This was great back when stress meant a charging saber-toothed tiger or an attacking horde of barbarians, and you could turn and head for the hills. But you can't really run away from a deadline or take up arms against a traffic jam. All you can do is bear down and, to help soothe your nerves, maybe have a snack. And another. Meanwhile, a second hormone called cortisol grabs all those fatty acids from your bloodstream and stores them in your belly region. With that fat stored, not burned, your body goes looking for more calories to replace the fatty acids it released earlier (back when it thought the hordes were invading).

Next time the pressure gets the best of you, brew a pot of black tea. Research found that the beverage can increase the rate at which your body is able to calm down and bring its cortisol levels back to normal. Although scientists are unsure what ingredient in the tea helps people bounce back, their findings are sound.

THE BLUBBER BLOCKER
BARBERRY

DRINK THIS: TerraVita, TeaHaven

BECAUSE IT: Prevents fat cells from growing larger

The stem, fruit, and root bark of the barberry shrub contain berberine–a powerful, naturally occurring, fat-frying chemical. A study conducted by Chinese researchers revealed that berberine can prevent weight gain and the development of insulin resistance in rats consuming a high-fat diet. Previous studies have also found that consuming the plant can boost energy expenditure and help decrease the number of receptors on the surface of fat cells, making them less apt to absorb incoming sources of blubber. Sounds like a good reason to have another cup of tea to me!

THE FAT CELL STOPPER
ROOIBOS

DRINK THIS: Celestial Seasonings, Teavana

BECAUSE IT: Inhibits the formation of fat cells

This red, naturally sweet tea made from the leaves of the rooibos bush is a powerful fat melter. Rooibos, also known as the "red bush" plant, grows exclusively in the small Cederberg region of South Africa, near Cape Town. According to South African researchers, polyphenols and flavonoids found in the plant inhibits adipogenesis–the formation of new fat cells–by as much as 22 percent. What makes rooibos tea particularly good for your belly is a unique and powerful flavonoid called aspalathin. Research shows this compound can reduce stress hormones that trigger hunger and fat storage and are linked to hypertension, metabolic syndrome, cardiovascular disease, insulin resistance, and type-2 diabetes.

THE BELLY SHRINKER
PU-ERH

DRINK THIS: Numi Organic Tea, Uncle Lee's Tea
BECAUSE IT: Shrinks Your Fat Cells

Pu-erh is a fermented green tea from China that is dried and rolled into blocks—and will give the willies to anyone who saw *Midnight Express*. But the microbial fermentation that happens as part of the process seems to give pu-erh additional fat-melting mojo. Chinese researchers divided rats into five groups and fed them varying diets over a two-month period. In addition to a control group, there was a group given a high-fat diet with no tea supplementation and three additional groups that were fed a high-fat diet with varying doses of pu-erh tea extract. The researchers found that the tea significantly lowered triglyceride concentrations (potentially dangerous fat found in the blood) and belly fat in the high-fat diet groups. Although sipping the tea could have slightly different outcomes in humans, there's enough research surrounding green tea's overall effects to make this exotic spin-off worth exploring.

Chai and Mighty!
Enjoy a spiced mug of potent medicine.

Drinking regular tea is like watching *Iron Man*. Drinking chai is like watching *The Avengers*: All your favorite superheroes, gathered up into one heaping serving.

Chai is black tea that arrives in your belly with a posse. That posse is a collection of herbs and spices, all of which have their own superpowers, and can help you fight the battle for your health on numerous fronts. Chai improves immunity, fights inflammation, slows aging, and enhances cardiovascular functioning. Because chai is a blend of different elements, the best way to understand it might be to break it down into its main components: black tea, ginger, cardamom, cinnamon, fennel, clove, and black pepper.

BLACK TEA Can increase the rate at which your body is able to calm down and bring its cortisol levels back to normal. Less stress = less hunger/snacking. A 2007 study published in the journal *Psychopharmacology* found that black tea drinkers are better able to manage stress than their herbal-sipping counterparts.

GINGER Blocks several genes and enzymes in the body that promote bloat-causing inflammation. Ginger is a powerful muscle relaxant that helps reduce soreness brought on by exercise by as much as 25 percent. It can also help banish bloat. Researchers attribute ginger's health benefits to gingerols, compounds that are antioxidant, anti-inflammatory, antibacterial—and anti-disease. In fact,

studies suggest ginger may reduce symptoms of arthritis, improve cholesterol, and prevent cancer.

CARDAMOM
Per the USDA Nutrient Database, the spice has 3.2 grams of fiber in 2 tablespoons (and only 36 calories)—so it can help boost satiety and stabilize blood sugar.

CINNAMON
Can help control blood sugar and prevent diabetes. One study found that adding a teaspoon of cinnamon to a starchy meal is as effective as older generation diabetes drugs at stabilizing blood sugar and warding off insulin spikes.

FENNEL
According to a 2015 *Journal of Food Biochemistry* study, *Foeniculum vulgare*–better known as fennel–has major inflammation-fighting properties. While the U.S. National Institutes of Health has no stance on fennel's medicinal effectiveness, Germany's Commission E, an official government agency similar to the FDA that focuses on herbs, says that the plant can indeed be an effective flatulence fighter. (Anything that can fight flatulence is A–OK in my book.)

CLOVE
A 2014 study in the journal *Oncology Research* reported that clove extract inhibits tumor growth. The herb also has antibacterial, antifungal, and antiviral properties, helps digestion, and may even help with pain relief.

BLACK PEPPER
Recent studies suggest piperine, a powerful compound found in black pepper, has the profound ability to decrease inflammation and interfere with the formation of fat cells, resulting in a decrease in waist size, body fat, and cholesterol levels.

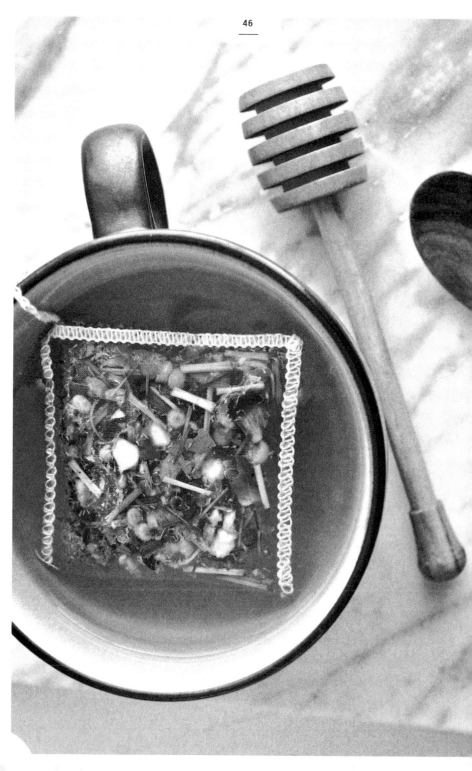

Metabolism-Boosting Teas

High-metabolism teas that will turn
your calorie-burning furnace
up a notch (or two!)

Think of your body as a teapot
on the stove, and think of the
water inside as your belly fat.
Chances are the pot is sitting
there over a low flame, not
doing much of anything.
The water inside may be warm,

METABOLISM-BOOSTING TEAS

but it's not boiling off. If you want the pot to whistle—and attract a few whistles yourself—you need to crank up the heat.

Well, that's exactly what will happen if you take that teapot from metaphor to reality by adding the teas in this chapter to your daily routine. Earlier in the book, we learned about teas that help stop weight gain by blocking the action of fat genes, inhibiting your body's ability to create new fat cells and literally starving your existing fat cells and forcing them to shrink.

It's powerful medicine, but it's only the first step in this full-body tea cleanse. In addition to preventing new fat cells from forming, certain types of teas can rev up your calorie burn as quickly and easily as turning a stove from low to high. Tea can reset your internal thermometer to increase metabolism and weight loss, in some cases by up to 10 percent, without exercising or dieting or sitting in a sauna dreaming about a Nestea plunge. Yup, sometimes the kettle can be as effective as the kettlebell.

Remember, any one of these teas can get the metabolism-boosting job done. Find one you like best, or try a different one each day!

THE FAT MELTER
GREEN TEA

DRINK THIS: Lipton, Yogi
BECAUSE IT: Unlocks your fat cells

Before a workout, crank your metabolism up from Bach to Beyoncé and turbocharge the fat-blasting effects of exercise by sipping a cup of green tea. In a recent 12-week study, participants who combined a daily habit of four to five cups of green tea each day with a 25-minute sweat session lost an average of 2 more pounds than the non-tea-drinking exercisers. Once again it's the power of the unique catechins found in green tea that can blast adipose tissue by triggering the release of fat from fat cells (particularly in the belly), and then speed up the liver's capacity for turning that fat into energy.

THE POUND-A-WEEK SHREDDER
OOLONG TEA

DRINK THIS: Bigelow, Stash
BECAUSE IT: Boosts metabolism

Oolong, a Chinese name for "black dragon," is a light, floral tea that, like green tea, is also packed with catechins, which help promote weight loss by boosting your body's ability to metabolize lipids (fat). A study in the *Chinese Journal of Integrative Medicine* found that participants who regularly sipped oolong tea lost 6 pounds over the course of the six-week time period. That's a pound a week!

METABOLISM-BOOSTING TEAS

THE EXERCISE EXTENDER
YERBA MATÉ

DRINK THIS: Guayaki Organic, Mate Factor

BECAUSE IT: Makes your fat burners more sensitive to exercise

This tea is known for its powerful thermogenic effects—meaning it turns up your body's calorie-burning mechanism—and can also promote weight loss by improving insulin sensitivity. In a recent study, participants were divided into two groups. One group took a placebo 60 minutes prior to exercising, while the other group ingested a 1,000mg capsule of yerba maté. Researchers found that those who consumed the herb increased the beneficial effects their workouts had on their metabolism.

THE CALORIE CONSUMER
GOJI

DRINK THIS: Stash, The Republic of Tea

BECAUSE IT: Cranks up calorie burn by 10 percent

Dried goji berries might be a staple of every health food store, but it's worth looking for them a couple of aisles over in the tea section. *Lycium barbarum*, the plant from which gojis are harvested, is a traditional Asian medicinal therapy for diabetes and other diseases, but it also boasts a slimming effect. In a study published in the *Journal of the American College of Nutrition*, participants were given either a single dose of L. barbarum or a placebo after a meal. The researchers found that one hour after the dose, the goji group was burning calories at a rate 10 percent higher than the placebo group. The effects lasted up to four hours. Bonus: Most goji teas are mixed with green tea, further boosting your calorie burn.

THE FAT-BURNING BUZZ SAW
KOLA NUT

DRINK THIS: Celestial Seasonings, Yogi Vital Energy
BECAUSE IT: Boosts metabolism with a single cup

Clocking in at caffeine counts higher than a cup of coffee, these teas are sure to zap any morning drowsiness–and set your metabolism up for a hotter burn. In a study published in the journal *Physiology & Behavior*, a 3 to 4 percent increase in metabolic rate was measured in both lean and obese subjects after a single 100-milligram dose of caffeine. Look for teas made from this caffeine-containing fruit. If you want to skip the label reading, just grab a box of Celestial Seasoning's Fast Lane, which clocks in 20-milligrams above your daily cup of coffee at 110 milligrams caffeine.

Kombucha Con?

Why this home-brewed tea drink might cause more worries than it's worth.

If you follow food trends—or if you live in a place like Brooklyn, Austin, Portland or other centers of hipster culture—you've probably heard a lot about Kombucha tea. And you're probably wondering, How come it's not part of *The 7-Day Flat-Belly Tea Cleanse*?

Otherwise known as Manchurian tea, Kargasok tea, or, less glamorously, "tea fungus," kombucha is a fermented drink made from tea, sugar, bacteria and yeast. Although it's sometimes referred to as kombucha mushroom tea, kombucha isn't a mushroom—it's a colony of bacteria and yeast. Brewers add sugar and tea—usually black tea—to the colony and allow the mix to ferment; the resulting liquid tastes a lot like sparkling apple cider and contains vinegar, B vitamins and a number of other chemical compounds.

Proponents claim that kombucha can stimulate the immune system (specifically by increasing T-cell count), prevent cancer, bolster cognition, aid weight loss, and improve gut health. As a result, kombucha enthusiasts promote it as a cure-all for a wide range of conditions, from the major (HIV, MS, and cancer) to the minor (hair loss, insomnia, indigestion).

You know where this is going: When a product is said

to cure everything, it seldom actually cures anything. In fact, there are no studies on humans that show kombucha promotes good health, prevents any ailments, or works within the body to cure cancer or any other ailment. One small pilot study did find that mice that sipped kombucha tended to live longer, and other small animal studies have shown some benefits. But remember, kombucha is made from black tea. It's likely that any health benefits that are eventually found can be attributed to that key ingredient.

And as for the big colony of yeast and bacteria you're enjoying? Kombucha's popularity is in part due to the probiotics found in the tea, which are similar to those found in yogurt or kefir; however, most commercially available kombuchas are pasteurized, which destroys all bacteria, good, bad, and in between. Unpasteurized kombucha drinks have been linked to bacterial infections, allergic reactions, and liver damage. Women who are pregnant or breast-feeding should not drink kombucha, according to several medical organizations.

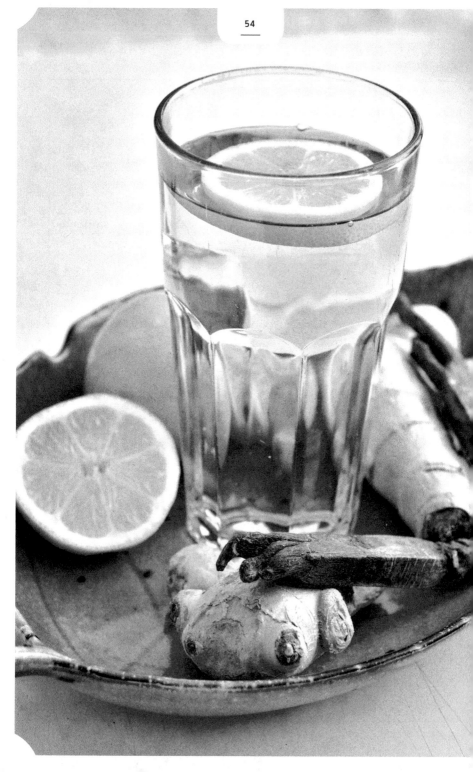

Flat-Belly Teas

End bloat, calm inflammation
and set your body on
a crash course to leanness

Bloating, gas, hunger pangs,
cravings—they're all signs
that something's amiss in your
midsection. And while most
of us think of such issues
as annoying and embarrassing,
they're actually something

more: signs that your body is in fat-storage mode.

See, digestive issues typically signal that there's an imbalance in your gut health. It can be brought on by too much bad food (or not enough good food, especially fiber-packed options), which feeds the bad bacteria and starves the good guys; or by too much stress, which cranks up the stomach acids. Either way, an upset stomach and the bloating that go with it aren't harmless. Bloating means inflammation in your digestive tract, and inflammation leads to weight gain by stressing your system and causing it to store fat. In a study published in the *British Journal of Nutrition* in 2013, researchers looked at overweight women and men who were put on a calorie-restrictive diet and given either a placebo or a probiotic supplement for 12 weeks. At the end of the 12 weeks, women who had received the healthy probiotic showed significantly greater weight loss than those who had the placebo. Even more impressive, the treatment was then stopped and the subjects measured again 12 weeks later. The women who had rebalanced their guts kept losing weight, even after the study ended.

And not only will you lose weight steadily, you'll lose weight suddenly and surprisingly. According to the American Society for Clinical Nutrition, a healthy bug called L. plantarum, found in plant-based foods like tea, can decrease bloating. That means you'll look and feel considerably slimmer in just days. To reap the maximum benefits, you'll need to sip a tea variety that either fights back against stomach-swelling inflammation, reduces water retention, or helps keep food cravings at bay. These brews are your best bets. Any one of them will do the job, so if you have a favorite, simply stick with it each day. Or buy a variety and see which appeals most to you!

THE CRAVINGS CRUSHER
MINT TEA

DRINK THIS: Tazo, Teavana
BECAUSE IT: Wards off the munchies

Fill a big teacup with soothing peppermint tea, and sniff yourself skinny! While certain scents can trigger hunger (a trick Cinnabon figured out long ago), others can actually suppress your appetite. One study published in *The Journal of Neurological and Orthopaedic Medicine* found that people who sniffed peppermint every two hours lost an average of 5 pounds a month. (Although tea is relatively low in caffeine—about 25 percent of what a cup of coffee delivers—decaffeinated varieties are great to have on hand for a soothing bedtime treat.) In a similar study in the journal *Appetite*, those who sniffed peppermint consumed 2,800 fewer calories a week. (At that rate, you'd drop a shocking 41½ pounds in a year—just by sipping and sniffing peppermint!) To further mellow out your cravings, consider also adding a few drops of peppermint oil to your pillow or burning a minty candle to fill the room with slimming smells.

THE BELLY BANISHER
GINGER TEA

DRINK THIS: Bigelow, Tazo, Yogi
BECAUSE IT: Reduces stomach irritation

If the flat stomach you saw in the mirror before hitting the sheets seems to have vanished overnight, inflammation–often brought on by spicy foods, dairy and chemical additives–may be to blame. According to numerous studies, ginger, traditionally used to ease stomach pain, blocks several genes and enzymes in the body that promote bloat-causing inflammation. If you prefer the taste of chai tea (typically made from a blend of cinnamon, cardamom, cloves, and ginger), that may also do the trick—but may be less potent.

THE INFLAMMATION ENFORCER
BILBERRY TEA

DRINK THIS: Alvita, Celebration Herbals
BECAUSE IT: Ends inflammation

Consuming bilberries, a northern European cousin to the blueberry, may help reduce bloat-inducing inflammation according to *Molecular Nutrition & Food Research*. To come to these findings, researchers divided participants into two groups. One group was given a diet that included an equivalent of 1.5 cups of blueberries, while the other group followed a control diet that didn't include the fruit. At the end of the experiment, the bilberry-eating group had significantly less inflammation than their counterparts who didn't munch on the berries. Since the fruit is native to northern Europe, it isn't widely available in the U.S. To reap the benefits, enjoy a few cups of bilberry tea. I'm willing to bet the results will be similar.

THE FLUID FIXER
HIBISCUS

DRINK THIS: Alvita, Bigelow, Good Nature
BECAUSE IT: Activates your flat-belly hormones

One day your jeans fit, the next it seems like Kate Moss snuck in and stuck her pair in your dresser. Breathe easy: You didn't actually pack on the pounds. Your new paunch is likely a result of eating some salty foods or hormonal fluctuations—both scenarios can cause the body to store sodium and fluids. Luckily, science has a solution: According to numerous studies, flavonoids and other compounds found in the hibiscus plant help to counteract bloating by influencing how aldosterone, the hormone that regulates water and electrolytes balance, affects the body. Enjoy a cup of hibiscus tea and watch your pooch slowly–but surely–deflate.

THE TUMMY SOOTHER
FENNEL TEA

DRINK THIS: Alvita, Traditional Medicinals
BECAUSE IT: Deflates the gas

According to a 2015 *Journal of Food Biochemistry* study, *Foeniculum vulgare*–better known as fennel–has major inflammation-fighting properties. Fans of the mild, sweet licorice-flavored tea have long used it to treat gas and other gastrointestinal issues, too. While the U.S. National Institutes of Health has no stance on fennel's medicinal effectiveness, Germany's Commission E, an official government agency similar to the FDA that focuses on herbs, says that the plant can indeed be an effective flatulence fighter.

THE BLOAT BUSTER
LEMON TEA

DRINK THIS: Bigelow, Celestial Seasonings, Lipton
BECAUSE IT: Shrinks the bloat

Next time you're feeling big as a blimp, burst the bloat with a hot cup of lemon tea. What makes it so powerful? D-limonene, the major component of citrus-rind oil, is commonly found in the brew. The extract has been used for its diuretic effects since ancient times, but until recently there were no scientific findings to back the assumption. A recent animal study published in the *Journal of the Pharmaceutical Society of Japan* confirmed D-limonene can indeed fight off water retention.

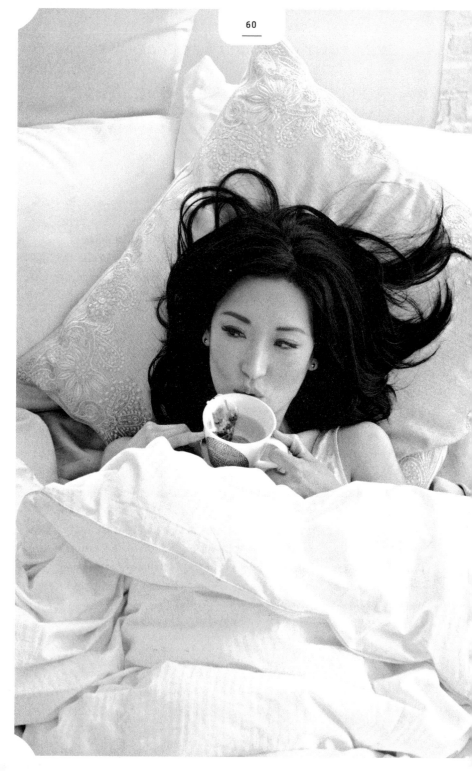

Stress-Busting Teas

Discover how the right teas
will ease your days and bring calm,
restful sleep back to your nights

What if I told you that the biggest contributor to your weight gain wasn't sugary drinks, or too much couch time, or the 1,800-calorie Bloomin' Onion you ate the last time you visited Outback?

What if the real culprit was something more sneaky and insidious, something you couldn't see, couldn't taste, and couldn't get out of your life? No, I'm not talking about the Kardashians. I mean something even more ubiquitous: stress.

Stress causes fat gain in several different ways:

The stress-nosh effect.
You're anxious/bored/worried/tired, and you need something to occupy your hands/your mouth/the empty feeling in your gut, so you automatically reach for a cookie/brownie/slice of cake/entire bag of Doritos. Stress drives us to distraction, and distracted eating is eating that adds a lot more calories but little, if any, quality nutrients or feelings of satisfaction.

The fat-storage effect.
When you're under stress, the hormone cortisol gathers up all the extra lipids in your bloodstream and stores them right in your belly. Then it sends out a signal: "Hey, need more lipids here. Go eat something." More stress leads to more belly fat, even if actual calories consumed remain the same.

The sleeplessness effect.
Sitting up all night long because you can't stop thinking about your credit report, your kids' school report, or how much you miss *The Colbert Report* may set you up for a miserable day of nutrition. A study in *The American Journal of Clinical Nutrition* found that when people are sleep-deprived, they are more likely to make bad food choices, snack late at night, and choose high-carb snacks. And a second study found that when people miss out on shut-eye, it makes them eye more calorie-dense meals.

That's why using tea to battle stress is an important part of *The 7-Day Flat-Belly Tea Cleanse*. The following teas can help soothe the soul, bring calm and focus to your world, and improve the quality of your sleep, even on evenings when the gap between income in and payments out is looking precariously narrow. Choose any of the below, or buy yourself a variety and experiment with a different one each night!

THE SLEEP ENHANCER
VALERIAN TEA

DRINK THIS: Yogi Tea Herbal Tea Supplement, Bedtime
BECAUSE IT: Brings on deeper sleep

Valerian is an herb that's long been valued as a mild sedative, and now research is showing what tea enthusiasts have known for centuries. In a study of women, researchers gave half the test subjects a valerian extract and half a placebo. Thirty percent of those who received valerian reported an improvement in the quality of their sleep, versus just 4 percent of the control group. In a study published in the *European Journal of Medical Research*, investigators gave 202 insomniacs valerian or a Valium-like tranquilizer. After six weeks, both treatments were equally effective. And in other studies, valerian root has been shown to increase the effectiveness of sleeping pills. While researchers have yet to identify the exact active ingredient, they suspect that receptors in the brain may be stimulated to hit "sleep mode" when coming in contact with valerian.

THE BLUES BUSTER
CHAMOMILE & LAVENDER TEA

DRINK THIS: Traditional Medicinals Organic Chamomile with Lavender
BECAUSE IT: Reduces fatigue and depression

Here's the funny thing about chamomile: While it's the most popular tea for bedtime, there's actually no evidence that it improves the length or quality of sleep. But there's a lot of evidence that it does something even more mysterious: It reduces the stress that comes with insomnia. One German study found that chamomile tea significantly improved the physical symptoms related to a lack of sleep and even helped reduced levels of depression in the chronically sleep-deprived. Another study found that it improved daytime wakefulness in people who suffered from a lack of sleep. To maximize its effects, look for a chamomile/lavender blend. In a study of postpartum women, those who drank lavender tea for 2 weeks showed improvement in postpartum depression and reduced fatigue. They also reported being able to better bond with their infant.

THE INSOMNIA SLAYER
LEMON BALM

DRINK THIS: Traditional Medicinals Organic Lemon Balm
BECAUSE IT: Reduces sleep disorders

A European study found that lemon balm serves as a natural sedative, and researchers reported that they observed reduced levels of sleep disorders among subjects using lemon balm versus those who were given a placebo.

THE NERVE SOOTHER
HOPS

DRINK THIS: Celestial Seasonings Tension Tamer
BECAUSE IT: Reduces anxiety

The hop, a component in beer, is a sedative plant whose pharmacological activity is due primarily to the bitter resins in the leaves. Hops increase the activity of the neurotransmitter gamma-aminobutyric acid, or GABA, which soothes the central nervous system. Spanish researchers reported in a 2012 journal report that the sedative activity of hops aids nocturnal sleep.

THE STRESS-HORMONE SQUASHER
ROOIBOS

DRINK THIS: Celestial Seasonings, Teavana
BECAUSE IT: Reduces cortisol levels

What makes rooibos tea particularly good for soothing your mind is the unique flavanoid called aspalathin. Research shows this compound can reduce stress hormones that trigger hunger and fat storage and are linked to hypertension, metabolic syndrome, cardiovascular disease, insulin resistance, and type-2 diabetes.

THE ANXIETY STOPPER
PASSIONFLOWER

DRINK THIS: Yogi Tea Herbal Tea Supplement, Bedtime
BECAUSE IT: Induces sleepiness and aids anxiety

Passionflower has the flavone chrysin, which has wonderful anti-anxiety benefits and, in part, can work similarly to the pharmaceutical Xanax (alprazolam). A mild sedative, this particular species of passionflower provides a vegetal-tasting tea that calms nervousness and anxiety and helps you get to sleep at night. It is generally considered safe to use but should be avoided by pregnant women.

THE PERSPECTIVE CHANGER
ASHWAGANDHA

DRINK THIS: Yogi Tea Herbal Tea, Sweet Tangerine Positive Energy
BECAUSE IT: Gives you a better outlook on life

A study in the *Indian Journal of Psychological Medicine* found that "ashwagandha root extract safely and effectively improves an individual's resistance towards stress and thereby improves self-assessed quality of life." In another study, serum-cortisol levels in a group of ashwagandha drinkers were substantially reduced versus a placebo group. The plant is used in traditional ayurvedic medicine to treat nervous exhaustion, insomnia, and loss of memory.

THE MIND QUIETER
KAVA KAVA

DRINK THIS: Yogi Tea Herbal Tea, Kava Stress Relief
BECAUSE IT: Quells worrying thoughts

It's one thing to simply sedate. But unlike other teas studied, kava kava actually reduces anxiety levels by helping you get a healthier perspective on life. In one study, 120 milligrams of kava kava was administered daily over six weeks to patients who had stress-induced insomnia. The results suggested a statistically significant improvement in sleep latency, duration, and waking mood. A 2010 study out of Melbourne found its efficacy so impressive that the Kava Anxiety-Lowering Medication (KALM) project was established to lobby for its reintroduction. Note: At very high levels, kava kava can cause liver toxicity; it should be only one part of an overall balanced tea cleanse.

All Your Worries Solved—With Tea!

"Let food be thy medicine"
—Hippocrates

Food is medicine, and drink maybe even more so. When you set a pot to boil on the stove, you're calling up some serious medical support, stat. Besides the weight-loss and health properties you'll read about in the coming pages, some teas have other magical properties that can do everything from focus your mind to fry your anxiety. Here's the right tea to drink...

When You're Stressed:
PEPPERMINT TEA

Researchers in Cincinnati found that it took a mere whiff of peppermint to increase subjects' concentration and performance on tedious tasks, and a professor in West Virginia claimed that he used the magical herb to improve athletes' performance and focus. In another study, researchers found that peppermint makes drivers more alert and less anxious.

When You've Had Too Much to Drink:
GREEN TEA

A study published in the journal *Biological Chemistry* showed that green tea protected the liver from some of the oxidative stress brought on by alcohol.

When Everyone Around You Is Sick:
GINSENG TEA, hot or iced

In a Canadian study, people who took 400 milligrams of ginseng a day had 25 percent fewer colds than those popping a placebo. Ginseng helps kill invading viruses by increasing the body's production of key immune cells.

When You Feel the Sniffles Coming On:
GREEN TEA

EGCG, a chemical compound that is potent in green tea, has been shown to stop the adenovirus (one of the bugs responsible for colds) from replicating. Start pumping green tea into your system at the first sign of a cold and you should be able to stave off worse symptoms. The best brand to brew? Go with Tetley; it was the most effective brand in studies.

When a Cold Has You in Its Grasp:
ROOIBOS TEA with honey

Preliminary studies have shown that rooibos, a red tea from South Africa, may have the same kickstart effects on your immune system as green tea. But with its richer flavor, rooibos will help cut through the dulled senses that come with a stuffy nose. And to keep your symptoms in check, drizzle in a little honey: Penn State scientists have discovered that honey is a powerful cough suppressant. When parents of 105 sick children doled out honey or dextromethorphan (the active ingredient in over-the-counter cough medicines like Robitussin), the honey was better at lessening cough frequency and severity.

When the Sushi Looks Sketchy:
ANY TEA

Worried about all the scary blog posts about contaminants in seafood? Purdue University researchers found that drinking tea with dinner may block the absorption of any toxins in your tuna. (In fact, if you're worried about toxins like mercury, then get to know your tuna: light chunk tuna is lower in mercury content than albacore.) Other low-mercury seafood include shrimp, wild salmon, pollock, and catfish. Avoid higher-contaminant fish like Atlantic salmon, swordfish, shark, king mackerel, marlin, and tilefish.

When You Had a Tough Workout:
GREEN TEA

Brazilian scientists found that participants who consumed three cups of the beverage every day for a week had fewer markers of the cell damage caused by resistance to exercise. That means that green tea can help you recover faster after an intense workout.

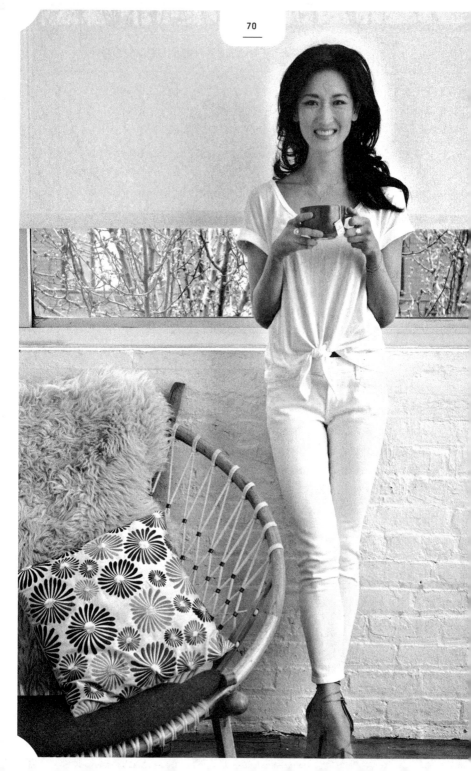

The Tea Cleanse Food Plan

A complete eating plan incorporating your teas with delicious foods that strip away fat, fast

On *The 7-Day Flat-Belly Tea Cleanse*, you'll most likely see significant results within just the first 72 hours. People who have tried it report losing up to 3 inches from their waists in just one week.

THE TEA CLEANSE FOOD PLAN

The Tea Cleanse is a plan for perfect eating, albeit an intense one, which is why I'm not recommending you make it a routine for more than seven days. But during the next week, you're also going to learn some amazing things about your body and how easily and quickly you can teach it to strip off unwanted fat automatically. And you'll be able to return to this seven-day plan whenever you have a big event coming up, just the way you crammed during finals week to pass Applied Calculus. Here's what the plan looks like:

TEAS

You'll enjoy one cup of tea, five times a day, during the cleanse. Each is carefully selected to provide your body with the maximum benefits it needs at the very time that it needs it.

- One to two metabolism-boosting teas to rev up your fat burners

- One flat-belly tea to fight inflammation and reduce bloating

- Two weight-loss teas (before lunch and dinner) to shrink your fat cells, prevent weight gain and reduce hunger

- One stress-busting tea to reduce anxiety, improve focus and ensure better sleep

WHY IT WORKS: A balanced diet means exactly that: You're finding a proper balance of all the nutrients your body needs in a day. Because each tea has its own particular set of special properties, I've balanced the four key types of tea to ensure your body gets everything it needs each and every day.

MEAL PLAN

One Tea Cleanse smoothie for lunch, a delicious Tea Cleanse dinner, and no dessert. (Hey, it's only a week! I'll explain more about the dessert embargo, below.)

WHY IT WORKS: The average American woman consumes between 1,850 and 2,200 calories every day; the average American man, closer to 2,700. This cleanse brings your daily calorie intake to about 1,000. That calorie deficit alone means the average woman will drop 4 pounds in 10 days just on calories alone—and the average man, about 5. But that's before factoring in the metabolic impact, the debloating power, and the way in which teas cause fat cells to resist growth. According to the latest research, your results may be as much as 14 pounds in seven days!

TEA SMOOTHIES

Every day, you're going to look forward to enjoying a cool, creamy and delicious tea smoothie at lunchtime. Just like the smoothies you love from places like Jamba Juice or Smoothie King, these blended drinks are a delicious blast of sweet, soothing nutrition. But unlike those joints, these smoothies will do something very different: They'll strip fat from your body instead of packing it on with obscene sugar counts. Consider this:

At Smoothie King, a 20-ounce Peanut Power Plus Chocolate will cost you 698 calories and 63 grams of sugar. (That's as much sugar as you'll find in 10 chocolate Oreos!) And an Orange Ka-Bam packs 469 calories and 108 grams of sugar. (That's what you'd get from 43 gummy bears!)

At Jamba Juice, a Strawberry Surf Rider will cost you 450 calories and 98 grams of sugar. (That's 3 full cups of Breyers Vanilla Ice Cream!)

At Starbucks, an Iced White Chocolate Mocha delivers 340 calories and 52 grams of sugar. (That's like having 3½ Snicker's Ice Cream Bars!)

WHY IT WORKS: Tea Cleanse Smoothies are carefully balanced to provide you with all the nutrition your body needs in a super-low-calorie drink, and they use the added punch of green tea to make sure your metabolism keeps revving.

CLEANSE FOODS

Tell your friends that your weekly dinner at Cracker Barrel is canceled for this week. To make the cleanse work for you, you'll need to make your own dinners for the next seven days, or special order off the menu of your favorite restaurant. Tea Cleanse dinners are under 500 calories, and consist of protein and vegetables, healthy fats, and limited amount of grains and fruits. A little harsh, but again, it's only temporary.

WHY IT WORKS: Metabolism decreases up to 35 percent during sleep. That means that any extra carbs in your system at bedtime are more likely to get converted to glucose, and then stored as fat. Grains and fruit are the two main sources of carbohydrates in the American diet.

ALCOHOL

No more than one drink every other day, preferably wine.

WHY IT WORKS: For starters, alcohol is loaded with calories, so cutting down on booze is one of the fastest ways to get rid of empty calories. But alcohol is particularly bad for your weight because it's a toxin. Ingest a beer or a glass of wine and your body mobilizes to burn off the calories in that drink as quickly as possible—ignoring any other calories that might have come along with it. So whether it's wine and cheese or beer and wings, the drink gets metabolized while the body shoves a higher percentage of the accompanying food calories into fat cells.

MORNING RITUAL

Every day, you'll start with a 10- to 30-minute walk to jump-start your metabolism.

WHY IT WORKS: More and more studies have shown that "fasted" exercise—meaning, a workout before your first meal of the day—is a more effective fat burner than exercise later in the day. The key is to do a light workout before you eat anything—no latte, no smoothie. The only thing to have beforehand is a metabolism tea, which will help maximize the effects of your workout. Here's why: Once you eat, you give your body a boost of glycogen—the energy that powers your day. So now when you go to exercise, you need to burn off that glycogen before you start to touch your fat stores. But walk before you eat, and your burn will come primarily from fat. A study from Northumbria University found that people burn up to 20 percent more body fat by exercising in the morning on an empty stomach.

DESSERT

None (for the next seven days, at least).

WHY IT WORKS: By ending your eating by 7 p.m., you'll set yourself up to begin burning fat first thing in the morning. Not just burning calories—burning fat. And your first morning cup—a metabolism tea that jump-starts your body's internal furnace—will double the effects of your simple fast. Every step you take, every move you make (sorry, Sting), you'll be burning fat.

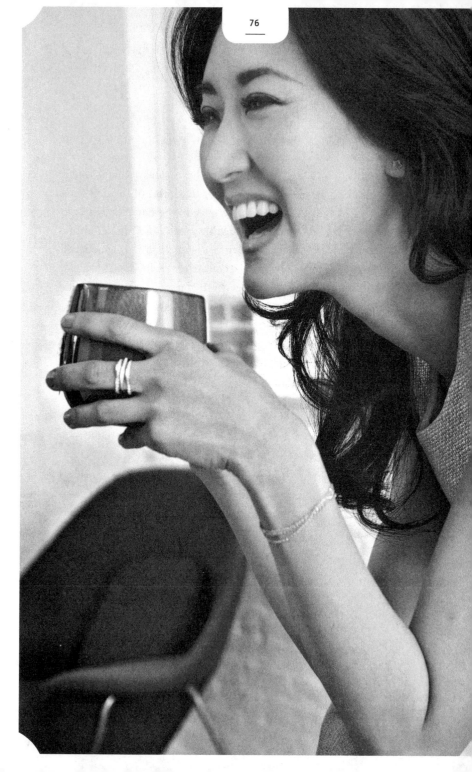

Frequently Asked Questions

1 *What if I didn't drink the number of teas as stated in your cleanse? Do I have to drink more the next day to make up for it?*

No. *The 7-Day Flat-Belly Tea Cleanse* is designed to optimize every single day, making each 24-hour period a perfect day of weight loss. But achieving perfection every day isn't realistic. Try to adhere as closely to the principles of the Tea Cleanse every day, and don't be too hard on yourself if you miss a few steps. There's always tomorrow!

2 Today was a particularly stressful day and I just couldn't resist the last few cookies in the box! What do I do?

Don't dwell on your binge. Everyone slips up sometimes. Next time you get a snack attack, though, reach for a tea that stops snacking: mint tea, green tea, and black tea all fit the bill for various reasons.

3 How long is my tea good for once I've opened it?

The most abundant green tea catechin, called epigallocatechin gallate, has been shown to decrease 28 percent during six months of storage in homelike conditions, while the second most abundant tea catechin decreased 51 percent. Thus, it's best to drink green tea as fresh as possible to enjoy the sensory and potential health benefits of these phytochemicals. Storing tea in sealed packaging in cool, dark conditions helps increase shelf life.

While fresh may be best for enjoying many types of teas, that's not always the case. Some pu-erh teas from China are considered to improve in taste with storage, much like a fine wine. In fact, the degradation and oxidation of catechins during storage of pu-erh teas result in the formation of new phytochemicals, which have come to be highly valued by tea drinkers for their rich, earthy taste and probiotic health properties.

4 What's better, tea bags or loose tea? Money's tight, and loose teas are pricey.

A report by ConsumerLab.com, an independent site that tests health products, found that green tea brewed from loose tea leaves was perhaps the best and most potent source of antioxidants like EGCG, though plain and simple tea bags made by Lipton and Bigelow were the most cost-efficient source. A single serving of Teavana's Gyokuro green tea, about 1 teaspoonful, was chock-full of antioxidants, yielding about 250 milligrams of catechins, a third of which were EGCG. A single bag of the green tea sold by Lipton and Bigelow contained somewhat smaller amounts of antioxidants than Teavana's green tea. But Teavana's recommended serving size was large, and the tea was also far more expensive, resulting in a higher cost per serving. The report calculated that the cost to obtain 200 milligrams of EGCG ranged from 27 cents to 60 cents with the tea bags, versus $2.18 with the Teavana loose tea leaves.

Tea brews made from loose leaf teas and tea bags did not differ appreciably in folic acid content, but tea bags can inhibit folic acid extraction.

So while loose leaves are the best, they're both more expensive and less convenient. Save them for special moments, and rest assured that your regular tea bag is doing more than enough to help turbocharge your weight loss.

5 I really don't have the time to measure the temperature of my water when I make tea. How much will temperature affect the taste and efficacy?

Just use hot water- don't get too caught up in the exact temps. In fact, simply taking a boiling kettle off the heat and letting it sit for 30 to 60 seconds before boiling should bring it right into the perfect range. But even cold water will work in a pinch, although you may need to let the tea steep longer.

6 I've heard most tea bags use toxins and harsh bleaches to dye them nice and white. Is it true? Is it dangerous?

Tea bags are made from a paper that is composed of wood and vegetable fibers. Oftentimes, this paper is bleached for appearance, and then the tea leaves and herbs are sealed inside using a thermoplastic material. There are a number of teas that market themselves as dioxin-, whitener-, and epichlorohydrin-free. However, in my extensive research, I couldn't find hard science or an official report that says there are any known downsides to standard tea bags. Most of the sources of this info weren't too reputable.

7 I know that tea contains oxalate, which some reports say can be harmful in large doses. How much oxalate am I getting on this cleanse?

Oxalate got a lot of attention in the spring of 2015 when one man fell ill from drinking massive amounts of tea, resulting in an oxalate intake of 1,500 mg per day. (He was drinking 16 large iced teas a day!) The Academy of Nutrition and Dietetics advises consuming no more than 40 to 50 milligrams of oxalate per day.

But even that number is hard to reach. While the amount of oxalate you receive from a cup of tea varies depending on the amount of tea in the bag and the steeping time, only black tea has significant levels of oxalate—and even then, you'd need to drink a lot of it to even approach hazardous levels. Here's how much oxalate you'll find in a typical cup of tea:

- Black tea: 1.36–12.6mg/cup
- Green tea: 0.23–4.36mg/cup
- White tea: 0.40–3.6mg/cup
- Oolong tea: 0.23–6mg/cup
- Herbal tea: In general, herbal teas have indetectable amounts of oxalate. Most go up to about 0.6mg per cup, max
- Rooibos: Indetectable amounts

So while you'll be drinking about 6 cups of tea a day on this cleanse (including the smoothies), only one cup—your daily black tea—has significant levels. As a result, the average daily oxalate content of the cleanse is about 13.25 milligrams a day. You'd probably need to drink four times as much tea in order to reach the top level of what's considered advisable! To be safe, though, be certain you're drinking black tea just once a day.

8 How do I store my teas? And how long are they really good for unopened?

EGCG, the active ingredient in green tea, is highly unstable under sunlight. Keep tea in a dark, dry place. Storing tea in sealed packaging in cool, dark conditions helps increase shelf life. If you brew iced tea, it will stay good for about four days, as long as you keep it refrigerated.

The long-term stability of green tea catechins like EGCG in canned and bottled drinks is currently unknown. What we do know is that store-bought, bottled teas typically lose 20 percent of EGCG/catechin content during the bottling process. If you really want bottled tea then shoot for versions with an acid like lemon juice or citric acid, which help stabilize EGCGg levels.

9 My iced tea seems to get cloudy after I brew it. Does that mean it's gone bad?

Not at all. The natural oil in the brewed tea will create cloudiness if you haven't cooled it to room temperature before refrigerating. Though it may not be very attractive, it's still fine to drink. If you've refrigerated tea too soon, and it has that slightly opaque look, just pour in some boiling water (1 cup per quart of iced tea) and stir to clear it.

Clouding is typically caused by the precipitation of the tannins in the tea. Stronger teas, and more high-quality teas, cloud faster because they have higher levels of tannins. Clouding can also be caused by minerals in your water, which are harmless. But if the effect bothers you, you may want to use a water filter.

10 What should I store my tea in?

I feel strongly about using glass, metal, or BPA-free plastic for storing tea. Tea is acidic, which means it's effective at leaching BPA (also known as bisphenol A) out of plastic containers. A 2011 Harvard study found that adults with the highest concentration of BPA in their urine had significantly larger waists and chances of being obese than those in the lowest quartile.

11 How is decaffeinated tea made? Is it harmful?

There are a number of ways tea may be decaffeinated. Up until the mid-1970s, all decaffeination was performed using organic solvents, until concerns about the side effects of solvents on both the body and the environment led the industry to find alternative methods. Here are the more common ones:

Ethyl acetate: One of the most common methods now used involves ethyl acetate, also known as acetic acid ethyl ester. Ethyl acetate is an ester and is a clear, volatile and flammable liquid, with a fruity flavor and a pleasant taste when diluted. Since it is found in many fruits, such as apples, peaches, and pears, and is completely digestible, it has been used in a wide range of foods, such as salad dressings and fruit desserts, and has been approved for decaffeination by the FDA since 1982.

Carbon dioxide: This is an ideal method with no toxic residues, less degradation of the tea catechins, and a high retention of the tea flavors. However, it's expensive to set up and not used as widely as it could be.

Water: Water decaffeination is done by first blanching freshly harvested green tea leaves in boiling water for a short period of time. Because the water solubility of caffeine is higher than the solubility of the tea catechins, most of the caffeine can quickly be extracted into the boiling water, whereas the catechins mostly remain behind in the tea leaves. The leaves are then quickly removed from the boiling water, which now contains the caffeine, and are then dried to obtain decaffeinated dried green tea.

12 I feel like I get jittery drinking all this tea. What do I do? I've lost a few pounds and I don't want to stop this cleanse.

Try to incorporate some decaf varieties. Many people avoid decaffeinated tea, believing that its beneficial properties are lost in the decaffeination process. However, the effect on polyphenols (the antioxidants) is considered to be marginal.

13 What is Fair Trade tea?

Fair Trade Certified tea comes from both cooperatives and large farms. Fair Trade helps tea farmers and workers gain access to capital, set fair prices for their products, and make democratic decisions about how to best improve their business, their community, and their tea.

Fair Trade certification protects tea estate workers as it ensures fair labor conditions and fair minimum wages. Fair Trade farmers gain access to international markets and are empowered to build organizational capacity to compete in the global marketplace. A minimum sales price is guaranteed to ensure a sustainable wage is paid to tea workers and a sustainable income is paid to tea farmers. All tea growers receive an additional Fair Trade premium to invest in their farms and communities. Fair Trade standards provide a framework for farms to increase their environmental sustainability.

14 Are tea bags reusable after one cup? After two?

A good tea will provide at least three infusions, but most of the important substances are extracted during the first infusion. So for maximum nutrient benefit, start with a fresh tea bag for each new cup.

However, if you are reusing a tea bag, you can boost antioxidant levels by adding a splash of vitamin C–rich juice such as lemon, orange, or pineapple to your cup. Studies on green tea showed that these juices help you absorb 13 times the amount of antioxidants.

It's Usually Someone Else's Fault...

Researchers from Eastern Illinois University have discovered that people consume 65 percent more calories when they eat with a person who opts for seconds than when they dine with a companion who doesn't. Instead of taking seconds, choose a cup of herbal tea after you finish your main course. It will keep your mouth busy while providing a refreshing, no-calorie end to your meal.

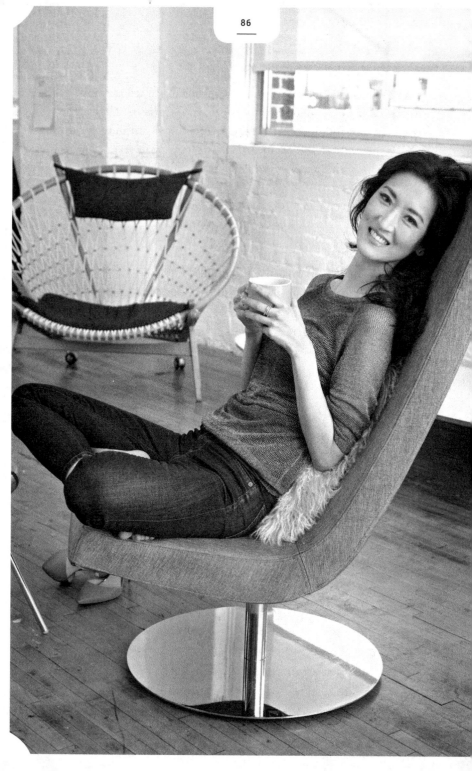

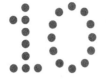

Superfoods to Boost Your Cleanse

Make sure your kitchen is stocked with the magic foods that make healthier living easy and weight-loss automatic

Combining *The 7-Day Flat-Belly Tea Cleanse* protocol with the recipes at the back of this book will give you all the nutrition you need to fuel your body day in and day out

SUPERFOODS

and drive toward maximum weight loss. But there are times when you want to add even more power to your diet regimen.

In those instances, consider reaching for one of these superfoods.

1 SPINACH

It may be green and leafy, but spinach is no nutritional wallflower. This noted muscle builder is a rich source of plant-based omega-3s and folate, which help reduce the risk of heart disease, stroke, and osteoporosis. It's also one of the 10 salad greens healthier than kale. Bonus: Folate also increases blood flow to the nether regions, helping protect you against age-related sexual issues. And spinach is packed with lutein, a compound that fights macular degeneration. Aim for 1 cup fresh spinach or ½ cup cooked per day.

FIT IT IN: Make your salads with spinach; add spinach to scrambled eggs; drape it over pizza; mix it with marinara sauce and then microwave for an instant dip.

2 YOGURT

Various cultures claim yogurt as their own creation, but the 2,000-year-old food's health benefits are not disputed: Fermentation spawns hundreds of millions of probiotic organisms that serve as reinforcements to the battalions of beneficial bacteria in your body. That helps boost your immune system and provides protection against cancer. Not all yogurts are probiotic, though, so make sure the label says "live and active cultures." Aim for 1 cup of the calcium and protein-rich goop a day. Much of the legwork to find the healthiest yogurt has already been done here, so all you have to do at the store is grab and go.

SUBSTITUTES: Kefir, soy yogurt

3 TOMATOES

There are two things you need to know about tomatoes: Red are the best, because they're packed with more of the antioxidant lycopene, and processed tomatoes are just as potent as fresh ones, because it's easier for the body to absorb the lycopene. Studies show that a diet rich in lycopene can decrease your risk of bladder, lung, prostate, skin, and stomach cancers, as well as reduce the risk of coronary artery disease. Aim for 22 milligrams of lycopene a day, which is about eight red cherry tomatoes or a glass of tomato juice.

SUBSTITUTES: Red watermelon, pink grapefruit, Japanese persimmon, papaya, guava.

FIT THEM IN: Pile on the ketchup and Ragú; guzzle low-sodium V8 and gazpacho; double the amount of tomato paste called for in a recipe.

4 CARROTS

Most red, yellow, and orange vegetables and fruits are spiked with carotenoids—fat-soluble compounds that are associated with a reduction in a wide range of cancers, as well as reduced risk and severity of inflammatory conditions such as asthma and rheumatoid arthritis—but none are as easy to prepare, or have as low a caloric density, as carrots. Aim for ½ cup a day.

SUBSTITUTES: Sweet potato, pumpkin, butternut squash, yellow bell pepper, mango

FIT THEM IN: Raw baby carrots, sliced raw yellow pepper, butternut squash soup, baked sweet potato, pumpkin pie, mango sorbet, carrot cake.

5 BLUEBERRIES

Host to more antioxidants than any other North American fruit, blueberries help prevent cancer, diabetes, and age-related memory changes (hence the nickname "brain berry"). Studies show that blueberries, which are rich in fiber and vitamins A and C, also boost cardiovascular health. Aim for 1 cup fresh blueberries a day, or ½ cup frozen or dried.

FIT THEM IN: Blueberries maintain most of their power in dried, frozen, or jam form.

6 BLACK BEANS

All beans are good for your heart, but none can boost your brain power like black beans. That's because they're full of anthocyanins, antioxidant compounds that have been shown to improve brain function. A daily ½-cup serving provides 8 grams of protein and 7.5 grams of fiber. Black beans are also low in calories and free of saturated fat.

SUBSTITUTES: Peas, lentils, and pinto, kidney, fava, and lima beans.

FIT THEM IN: Wrap black beans in a breakfast burrito; use both black beans and kidney beans in your chili; puree 1 cup black beans with ¼ cup olive oil and roasted garlic for a healthy dip; add favas, limas, or peas to pasta dishes.

7 WALNUTS

Richer in heart-healthy omega-3s than salmon, loaded with more anti-inflammatory polyphenols than red wine, and packing half as much muscle-building protein as chicken, the walnut sounds like a Frankenfood, but it grows on trees. Other nuts combine only one or two of these features, not all three. A serving of walnuts—about

1 ounce, or 7 nuts—is good anytime, but especially as a postworkout recovery snack.

SUBSTITUTES: Almonds, peanuts, pistachios, macadamia nuts, hazelnuts.

FIT THEM IN: Sprinkle on top of salads; chop and add to pancake batter; spoon peanut butter into curries; grind and mix with olive oil to make a marinade for grilled fish or chicken.

8 OATS

The éminence grise of health food, oats garnered the FDA's first seal of approval. They are packed with soluble fiber, which lowers the risk of heart disease. Yes, oats are loaded with carbs, but the release of those sugars is slowed by the fiber, and because oats also have 10 grams of protein per ½-cup serving, they deliver steady, muscle-friendly energy.

SUBSTITUTES: Quinoa, wild rice.

9 COCONUT OIL

One study from *The American Journal of Clinical Nutrition* found that subjects who ate coconut oil lost overall weight and belly fat faster than a group consuming the same amount of olive oil. The secret is in coconut's medium-chain triglycerides. Unlike the long-chain fatty acids in most oils, coconut oil is broken down immediately for use rather than stored and has been found to speed up metabolism. That's right—your body has trouble storing the calories in coconut oil and revs up its metabolism to burn them instead. Coconut oil's high smoke point makes it great for just about every dish from eggs to stir-frys and a delicious substitute for butter when baking.

10 FLAX AND CHIA SEEDS

One of the hallmarks of a balanced diet is to have a good ratio of omega-6 fatty acids to omega-3s. A 4-to-1 ratio would be ideal, but the modern American diet is more like 20-to-1. That leads to inflammation, which can trigger weight gain. But while eating a serving of salmon every day isn't exactly convenient, sprinkling these two seeds—among the most highly concentrated sources of omega-3s in the food world—into smoothies, salads, cereals, pancakes, or even desserts is as easy a diet upgrade as you can get. Animal studies suggest a chia-rich diet can lower harmful LDL cholesterol and protect the heart, and a recent study in the journal *Hypertension* found that daily consumption of flaxseed-fortified bakery products reduced blood pressure in patients with peripheral artery disease. Best absorbed when ground, flax adds delicious nuttiness to oats, cereal, smoothies and baked goods.

FIT THEM IN: Sprinkle 2 tablespoons ground flaxseed or chia seed on cereals, salads, and yogurt.

11 EGGS

Eggs are the single best dietary source of the B vitamin choline, an essential nutrient used in the construction of all the body's cell membranes. Two eggs will give you half your day's worth; only beef liver has more. (And believe me, starting your day with a slab of beef liver does not make for a great morning.) Choline deficiency is linked directly to the genes that cause the accumulation of belly fat. Eggs can solve the problem: Research has shown dieters who eat eggs for breakfast—as compared to a high-carb meal of a bagel—have an easier time losing weight due to their satiety value. At about 70 calories, a hard-boiled egg also makes an easy afternoon snack—just don't tell your coworkers. According to a personality analysis by the British

Egg Industry Council, boiled-egg consumers tend to be disorganized! (Other findings: fried-egg fans have a high sex drive and omelet eaters are self-disciplined.)

12 RED APPLES

A medium-size apple, at about 100 calories and 4.5 grams of fiber per fruit, is one of the best snack options for anyone looking to slim down—but especially apple-shaped folks. A recent study at Wake Forest Baptist Medical Center found that for every 10-gram increase in soluble fiber eaten per day, visceral fat (that's dangerous belly fat) was reduced by 3.7 percent over five years. Participants who paired their apple-a-day habit with 30 minutes of exercise two to four times per week saw a 7.4 percent decrease in the rate of visceral fat accumulation over the same time period. But don't peel your apple if you want to peel off the pounds: A study conducted at the University of Western Australia found that the blushing varieties (such as Pink Ladies) had the highest level of antioxidant phenols, most of which are found in the skin.

13 CINNAMON

It may be the easiest nutrition upgrade of all: Put cinnamon on your toast. According to researchers, cinnamon contains powerful antioxidants called polyphenols proven to improve insulin sensitivity and, in turn, our body's ability to store fat and manage hunger cues. A series of studies printed in *The American Journal of Clinical Nutrition* found that adding a heaping teaspoon of cinnamon to a starchy meal may help stabilize blood sugar and ward off insulin spikes.

14 AVOCADO

A scoop of guacamole is one of the most effective hunger squashers known to man. In a study published in *Nutrition Journal*, participants who ate half a fresh avocado with lunch reported a 40 percent decreased desire to eat for hours afterward. At only 60 calories, a 2 tablespoon serving of guacamole (on top of eggs, salads, grilled meats, etc.) can provide the same satiety benefit with even more of a flavor punch. Just be sure when buying store-bought guac that avocados actually made it into the container. (Many are made without the real fruit!) I love Wholly Guacamole as a store brand.

15 LETTUCE

Yep, lettuce. Move over, King Kale. In a new William Paterson University study that compared the 47 top superfoods by nutrient volume, the trendy superfood came in a respectable—but unremarkable—15th on the list. Ranking higher: watercress, spinach, leafy greens and endive. Make yourself a bowl of leafy greens and add some olive oil. According to a Purdue University study, as little as 3 grams of monounsaturated fat can help the body absorb vegetables' carotenoids (those magic molecules that protect you from chronic diseases like cancer and heart disease). Pairing your lettuce with a scant tablespoon of olive-oil-based vinaigrette is your best bet.

16 HUMMUS

A recent study published in the journal *Obesity* found that people who ate a single serving a day of garbanzo beans or chickpeas (which form the basis of hummus) each day reported feeling 31 percent fuller than their bean-less counterparts. Packed with fiber and protein, garbanzos have a low glycemic index, meaning that they break down slowly and keep you feeling full. The secret is to avoid varieties made with tahini; sourced from sesame seeds, tahini has a high omega-6-to-omega-3 fatty-acid ratio. Look for hummus that's olive-oil-based.

Eight Foods That Set Your Hormones at Ease

Depression. Bloating. Breakouts. Ugh. The side effects of PMS are just plain awful! If these or other nasty symptoms make you dread Mother Nature's monthly visit, you're not alone. According to the American College of Obstetricians and Gynecologists, more than 85 percent of women experience at least one uncomfortable premenstrual syndrome side effect.

The good news is that you don't have to live in misery or pop a pill to get relief every time your period comes around. Instead, take a walk to your kitchen (somewhere you were likely heading anyways, let's be honest) and whip up some symptom-slashing snacks. Believe it or not, there are a number of commonly consumed foods rich in the nutrients that help your body fight back against the wrath of your out-of-control hormones.

About to down that whole sleeve of cookies?
Toast up a piece of bread.

If every month, like clockwork, you get wild cravings for cookies and as emotional as you did the first time you watched *The Notebook*, you're not alone. The tears are flowing and your appetite is going wild because your serotonin (the mood-boosting, feel-good hormone) levels have dipped. Carb-rich foods (like those cookies calling you like a siren song) help to increase the amount of the hormone in your system. That's why those cravings are so hard to say no to—your body is hunting for a hormonal overhaul. Instead of caving to your inner Cookie Monster, turn to a healthy source of complex carbs like whole grain bread. The raisins in the Ezekiel 4:9 Cinnamon Raisin Sprouted Whole Grain Bread provide natural sweetness to nip your sugar craving in the bud while the vitamin B6- and manganese-rich whole grains help boost your mood. Toast up a slice as a midmorning mood-boosting snack.

Can't keep your hand out of the chip bag?
Pop some pumpkin seeds.

If you're cranky and seem to snap at the drop of a hat in the weeks leading up to your period, we can't say we blame you. PMS-ing is never a good time! The good news is, you can get through Mother Nature's visit without making your man wish he never put a ring on it. How? By munching on pumpkin seeds. The tiny yet powerful seeds may be able to ease your symptoms (and are likely the answer to your roommate's prayers). Just 1 ounce of the seeds serves up 75 percent of your day's magnesium, which can make you nicer and ward off water retention. (It's a win-win!) The nutrient can also help relax your blood vessels, nixing painful PMS headaches, too. Mix pumpkin seeds into your salads and veggie side dishes for a touch of crunch and some much-needed PMS relief.

Dreaming of death by chocolate?
Open up a can of beans. (Hear me out!)

Before I even get into their benefits, you should know this is leading to a brownie recipe. Beans are a magnesium–rich food that helps boost serotonin levels and diminish water retention. When choosing a can to prepare, stick with no–salt–added varieties. Sodium can make your body hold on to water, undermining the bean's bloat-busting effects. Bonus: These small but mighty seeds are antioxidant–rich and loaded with other good-for-you nutrients like iron, fiber, copper, zinc, and potassium. Add beans to salads, soups, or whole-grain pastas and rice dishes. Craving something more indulgent? Here it is, folks, the healthy bean brownies we promised: Blend 15 ounces of black beans and 1 cup of water together in a blender. Combine with a package of organic brownie mix, then combine until smooth. Bake in a greased baking dish for 25 minutes on 350 degrees F.

Craving movies and popcorn?
We give you permission to indulge.

Yes, you just read that right! Popcorn is a powerful PMS fighter for the same reason Ezekiel bread is beneficial— it's a whole grain that boosts the production of serotonin. Stick to unsalted varieties like Newman's Own Organics Unsalted Pop's Corn to keep salt-induced bloating at bay while simultaneously improving your mood. So go ahead, pop a fresh bag and turn on

Netflix. If there's any time you get a free pass to binge-watch *Scandal* guilt-free, it's this week.

Sporting a stubborn craving for Chunky Monkey?

Make a healthy variety at home.

In the weeks leading up to your period, do you speak without your edit button or turn into Cruella de Vil? If you said yes, that's totally okay. Luckily for you, if you're looking to reel it in a bit, we have a sweet suggestion: banana ice cream. A 2010 study of nearly 3,000 women published in *The Journal of Steroid Biochemistry and Molecular Biology* found that consuming calcium-rich dairy products with added vitamin D can lower the risk for nasty PMS symptoms by as much as 40 percent. Vitamin-D-fortified milk fits the nutritional bill. Although you may typically reach for skim milk because it's the lowest in calories, vitamin D is fat-soluble, which means you won't get all the benefits unless you opt for a variety with a bit of fat. Pour some into your morning oatmeal to reap the benefits all day long. Or if you're craving some Ben & Jerry's, try making our Banana Milk, a healthy spin on their classic Chunky Monkey (fudge chunks and walnuts not included, sorry). Simply blend a ripe banana with a half teaspoon of vanilla and a cup of milk, pour in a cup, and guzzle it down. Bonus: Bananas help fight PMS bloat.

Drowning your depression in donuts?
Fight the blues with a bit of yellow instead.

If during Mother Nature's monthly visit you typically feel so blue you want nothing more than to lie in a dark bedroom, we may have the cure you've been looking for: saffron. A *British Journal of Obstetrics and Gynaecology* study found that consuming the yellow-hued spice can significantly reduce PMS symptoms including feelings of depression. How? The spice increases serotonin levels, which typically drop before menstruation. Although saffron is one of the most expensive spices, a little of it goes a long way. Use it to whip up African-, Middle Eastern-, and European-inspired dishes and reap the PMS-busting benefits. The only caveat? You'll need to crawl out of bed to do your cooking, or cajole your significant other into whipping up dinner. (Just promise them you'll do the dishes.)

Dreaming of daiquiris?
Debloat with dressed-up melon.

Having a hard time buttoning those skinny jeans that just fit a couple of days ago? Breathe easy: You didn't gain weight! In the days leading up to your period, your body begins storing sodium and fluids. Instead of trading in your favorite pants for sweats and leggings, try munching on honeydew melon to debloat. Research suggests the fruit contains a compound called *Cucumis melo*, a diuretic that helps flush excess fluid from the body. That sugar-

and alcohol-filled daiquiri you're craving, however, does the opposite. The bottom line? Skip the fruity cocktail and stick with the fruit if you want to zip up your pants.

Instead of noshing on the fruit plain (boring!), make a mint, cilantro and melon salad. Here's how: Combine chunks of honeydew, fresh lime juice, chopped cilantro, mint and a touch of sugar in a bowl. Mix together, then enjoy.

Do you self-soothe with chocolate?
Try chia seeds instead.

Researchers think the nutrient may function like an antidepressant, although they aren't sure exactly which mechanisms are involved quite yet. Some researchers believe the nutrient makes it easier for serotonin to pass through the cell membranes, and in turn, this makes the effects of serotonin more powerful. While omega-3 can be found in salmon, enriched eggs, and grass-fed beef, I like chia seeds because they are portable and easy to pop into just about anything. Add the small but mighty seed into cereal, smoothies, and homemade baked goods to boost your intake and keep menstrual blues at bay.

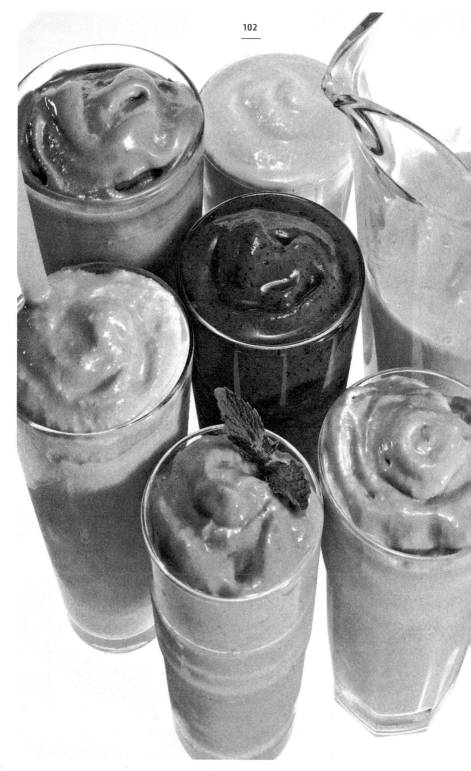

Tea Cleanse Smoothies

Weight-loss magic is just 90 seconds away

Unless you've been living in an igloo for the past two decades, you should know by now that Americans do not eat enough fruits and vegetables. In fact, recent surveys have found that only about 30 percent of Americans are eating the recommended 5 or more servings of fruits and vegetables a day. That's a pretty pitiful performance and no doubt a partial cause of the obesity epidemic that grips this nation.

If you happen to be one of those 7 out of 10 of us who don't eat enough plant matter, then you need to make fast friends with the smoothie. It's the quickest, most delicious way to make up for the fruit-and-vegetable deficit: Roll out of bed, toss some fruit in a blender, top with a bit of liquid, hit "liquefy." Boom! You're on the path to a skinnier, healthier existence.

Making smoothies can be a pretty freewheeling endeavor, which is certainly part of the fun, but we've established a few basic rules. Follow these and the ingredient-by-ingredient guide that follows and you'll be ready for liquid liftoff.

RULE 1
USE GREEN TEA AS YOUR BASE.

Because green tea has been shown to be so effective at attacking our fat-storage systems, and because its mild taste makes for a pleasant smoothie base (unlike harsher black teas), each of the recipes in this chapter uses the life-giving drink as a jumping-off point. Make a big pot of it and keep it chilling in your fridge for daily smoothie building.

RULE 2
ADD DAIRY.

I suggest half a cup of plain, low-fat or fat-free Greek-style yogurt (this will ensure that there is always adequate protein).

RULE 3
MAKE SURE YOU HAVE FIBER.

To slow digestion, keep you full, and ensure you're hitting your daily fiber content, consider adding a fiber booster like psyllium husk or flax meal.

RULE 4
BRING ON THE FRUIT.

Adding fruit to your daily smoothie helps to ensure that you're up to snuff on your vitamin intake. Your best weapon might be frozen fruit: Not only is it more affordable, but research has shown that frozen fruits may actually carry higher levels of antioxidants because they're picked at the height of the season and flash frozen on the spot. Also, frozen fruit means you can use less ice to make your smoothie sufficiently cold, which in turn yields a more intense, pure flavor. (Make sure the fruit is unsweetened.)

RULE 5
USE A STRONG BLENDER.

A weak blender won't be able to crush the ice quickly enough, which means it melts and ultimately dilutes your precious creation, rather than giving it that bracing, velvety texture you want.

RULE 6
RESPECT THE RATIO.

Once you learn the basic proportions of liquids to solids, you can turn anything into a pretty drinkable smoothie. For every 3 cups of fruit, you'll need about 1 cup of tea. Keep in mind that both yogurt and ice will thicken your drink.

SMOOTHIE SELECTOR

FRUIT

Nutritional info is for a 1-cup serving, unless otherwise stated.

MANGO
107 calories, 24 g sugars, 3 g fiber

This tropical treasure has become increasingly available in American supermarkets, in both fresh and frozen forms. Yes, it's higher in sugar than almost any other fruit in the produce section, but it also brings to the blender three-quarters of your day's vitamin C and 25 percent of your vitamin A. Consider added sweeteners entirely superfluous when making smoothies with mango.

PAPAYA
55 calories, 8 g sugars, 3 g fiber

Is there any fruit better for you than papaya? Flooded with vitamin C, replete with vision-strengthening vitamin A, and blessed with one of the most favorable fiber-to-sugar ratios imaginable, papaya proves itself to be one of the most well-rounded foods on the planet. Papaya also boasts papain and chymopapain, two potent enzymes that have been shown to fight inflammation, the cause of asthma, arthritis, and other serious conditions.

BLUEBERRIES
84 calories, 15 g sugars, 4 g fiber

Blueberries are best known in health circles for anthocyanins, the phytonutrients that give them their blue-red tint and their dense antioxidant punch. That punch translates into serious brain food, as blueberries have been found in studies to protect our noggins against both oxidative stress and the effects of age-related mental decay manifested in Alzheimer's and dementia.

STRAWBERRIES
49 calories, 7 g sugars, 3 g fiber

Beyond the monster dose of vitamin C (calorie for calorie, you'll get more C than you'd find in an orange), strawberries also prove to be a rich source of phenols, including the same brain-boosting, anti-inflammatory anthocyanins found in blueberries. They also lay claim to a rare and powerful antioxidant called ellagitannin, which has been shown to provide a stout defense against a variety of cancers.

BANANA *(1 medium)*
105 calories, 14 g sugars, 3 g fiber

Sure, there are fruits with deeper nutritional portfolios, but the humble banana serves as an all-star utility player in the smoothie game. Not only does it offer a handful of hard-to-find nutrients (heart-strengthening potassium, gut-friendly prebiotics), but it also provides smoothies with a balanced, creamy texture and enough natural sweetness to ensure no need for added sugar. Peel a few very ripe bananas, stick them in a plastic bag and toss them in the freezer. (Make sure you peel them before you freeze them, because the ice box turns their skins into little yellow Kevlar vests.)

AVOCADO *(1 medium Haas)*
227 calories, 21 g fat (3 g saturated), 9 g fiber

Avocado might not be a traditional smoothie constituent, but we're convinced that it should be. The calories come primarily from mono-unsaturated fat, the good stuff that protects your heart and helps beat back hunger. Add to that an impressive fiber load and you have the makings of a seriously satisfying smoothie. Plus, avocados add a richness that makes it feel like you're splurging, even when you're not.

PINEAPPLE
82 calories, 16 g sugars, 2 g fiber

Feeling low on energy? A cup of pineapple might just be the antidote. That's because pineapple is one of nature's best sources of manganese, a trace mineral that is essential for energy production. A cup provides 76 percent of your daily recommended intake, making pineapple nature's answer to Red Bull.

PEACH
60 calories, 13 g sugars, 2 g fiber

Peaches pack lutein and zeaxanthin, powerful carotenoids proven to help protect your peepers from macular degeneration. Plus, the blast of beta carotene may help stave off heart disease and cancer. But a USDA survey found that peaches are the most pesticide-laden fruit in the produce section, so if you can afford organic, you might want to spring.

THICKENERS & ENHANCERS

PEANUT BUTTER *(1 Tbsp)*

94 calories, 8 g fat (1.5 g saturated), 1 g sugars, 3.5 g protein

What's not to love about peanut butter? The fat is good for your heart, the protein is good for your muscles, and the package of vitamins and nutrients (vitamin E, manganese, niacin) will do plenty for the rest of your body. The only drawback is that peanut butter is extremely dense with calories (and don't bother with the reduced fat stuff—it's loaded with chemicals), so try to keep the quantity to no more than a tablespoon per smoothie.

FAT-FREE GREEK-STYLE YOGURT *(½ cup)*

70 calories, 0 g fat, 5 g sugars, 12 g protein

There may be no better addition to a smoothie than a healthy scoop of Greek yogurt. Not only does it give the smoothie a lovely body, but it also adds a ton of protein and gut-friendly bacteria to whatever concoction it graces. Why Greek? Because the Greeks are savvy enough to skim off the watery whey found in typical yogurt, thus yielding a creamier product with more than twice the protein found in the Dannons and the Yoplaits of the dairy world. Both Fage and Oikos are reliable brands found in most supermarkets. If you must stick to regular American-style yogurt, just make sure it's unflavored; opt for a fruit- or vanilla-flavored yogurt and you might as well be using ice cream.

HONEY *(1 Tbsp)*
64 calories, 0 g fat, 17 g sugars

As far as sweeteners go, honey ranks high on the list for the simple fact that it actually gives you something in return for all that sugar, namely a host of phytonutrients that have antiviral and antibacterial properties. Still, added sugar in any form is highly discouraged in the craft of smoothie making, so use honey sparingly, if at all.

FRESH MINT/FRESH BASIL *(2 Tbsp)*
2 calories, 0 g fat, 0 g sugars

Strange though it may sound, adding fresh herbs to smoothies is a small little trick that yields big results when properly employed. Plus, when you consider that fresh basil contains cancer-fighting carotenoids and that the menthol in mint can help facilitate easy breathing and relieve indigestion, what more motivation do you need? Basil pairs well with strawberries and watermelon, while mint works wonders on melon, blueberries, and papaya.

AGAVE SYRUP *(1 Tbsp)*
60 calories, 0 g fat, 15 g sugars

Let's be clear: As long as your smoothie is composed primarily of fruit, there is no reason to add sugar to the mix. But if you ever do reach for it, agave syrup is the way to go. The sweetness comes primarily from a form of fructose called inulin, which has a very gentle effect on your blood sugar, which not only helps prevent the dreaded sugar crash, but also keeps your body from going into fat storage mode. Score a bottle at most health food stores and grocers like Whole Foods.

BOOSTS

PROTEIN POWDER *(2 Tbsp)*
104 calories, 0 g fat, 16 g protein

No, protein powder isn't just for the muscle-mag set. Dozens of studies have highlighted the importance of getting protein first thing in the morning. Not only will it help to jolt your metabolism into action, it's also been shown to help you retain focus throughout the morning.

FIBER POWDER *(2 Tbsp)*
35 calories, 0 g fat, 9 g fiber

Often sold under the name of psyllium husk (for the seeds this powder is ground from), a dose of fiber is going to do more than promote a healthy colon. Fiber will slow the digestion of the smoothie in your stomach, which not only means you'll stay fuller longer, but also that the sugar from the fruit will have a less dramatic impact on your blood sugar levels. And if the Quaker Oats dude has taught us anything, it's that fiber promotes a healthy heart as well.

FISH OIL *(1 tsp)*
41 calories, 5 g fat (1 g saturated), 1,084 mg omega-3s

Fish oil has been canonized by hordes of wide-eyed nutritionists over the years, but the case for its sainthood sure is compelling. The tide of omega-3 fatty acids found in fish oil (usually made from fatty fish like salmon and sardines) may be the most versatile nutritional weapon out there, known to help protect the heart, fight inflammation, boost the brain, and reduce blood pressure, among other things. Look for a brand with a subtle flavor that will add all of the nutritional punch without leaving your smoothie tasting like a can of sardines. We like Carlson Fish Oil liquids.

GROUND FLAXSEED *(2 Tbsp)*
80 calories, 5 g fat (1 g saturated), 2,700 mg omega-3s

These seeds, picked and ground from the flax plant commonly found across the Mediterranean and Middle East, deliver a mother lode of omega-3s. Consider stirring them into your oatmeal or yogurt, but if you're looking for the easiest way to sneak flax into your diet, look to the blender for seamless integration.

WHEATGRASS POWDER *(1.25 Tbsp)*
35 calories

What doesn't wheatgrass offer? Even a tiny dose like this packs fiber, protein, tons of vitamin A and K, folic acid, manganese, iodine, and chlrophyll, to name a few. You don't need to know what each nutrient does for you; just know that a single tablespoon will have you operating at peak performance levels. Pick some up at amazinggrass.com.

Smoothie Recipes

The Green Banana

1 very ripe banana

½ cup green tea

½ cup milk

1 Tbsp peanut butter

1 Tbsp agave syrup

1 cup ice

With protein, healthy fat, and caffeine, this works perfectly as a start to your day or as a low-cal substitute for a milk shake.

311 calories, 52 g carbs, 10 g protein, 4 g fiber

The Purple Monster

1 cup blueberries

½ cup strawberries

½ cup green tea

½ cup Greek yogurt

3 or 4 cubes of ice

1 Tbsp flaxseed

Between the polyphenols in the blueberries and strawberries and the omega-3s in the flax, we're talking serious brain food.

248 calories, 42 g carbs, 16 g protein, 9 g fiber

___

The Orange Crush

¾ cup frozen mango
½ cup carrot juice
½ cup green tea
½ cup Greek yogurt
1 Tbsp protein powder
½ cup water

All that orange produce means this baby is stuffed full of vision-strengthening, cancer-fighting carotenoids.

218 calories, 42 g carbs, 13 g protein, 7 g fiber

___

Papaya Berry

¾ cup frozen papaya
¾ cup frozen strawberries
½ cup milk
½ cup green tea
1 Tbsp fresh mint

This is like a liquid mulitvitamin, loaded with vitamins A and C, plus disease-fighting carotenoids and lycopene.

250 calories, 52 g carbs, 16 g protein, 5 g fiber

___

Pineapple Punch

1 cup frozen pineapple
½ cup Greek yogurt
½ cup milk
½ cup green tea

Like a tropical island in a glass. In fact, a shot of rum would turn this into one heck of a healthy cocktail.

215 calories, 37 g carbs, 18 g protein, 4 g fiber

The Green Goddess

¼ avocado, peeled and pitted
1 ripe banana
1 Tbsp honey
½ cup green tea
1 scoop protein powder
½ cup ice
Optional: 1 tsp freshly grated ginger

Fiber and protein combine forces to vanquish any hunger in this untraditional, but tasty creation.

300 calories, 50 g carbs, 18 g protein, 6 g fiber

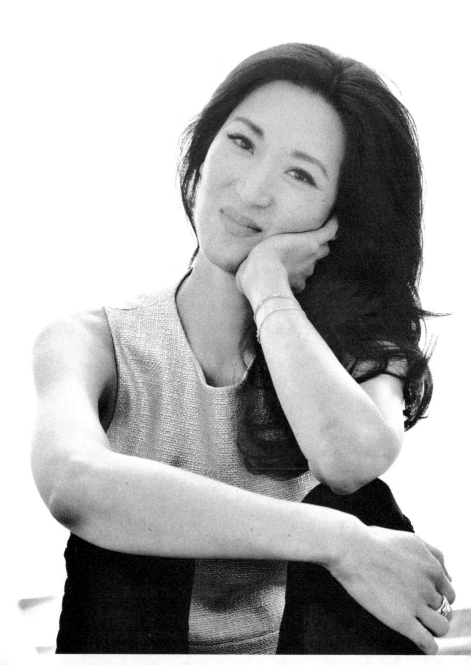

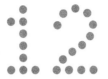

Tea Cleanse Food Plan & Recipes

Simple recipes that will boost your
Tea Cleanse success

Most "cleanses" are
pretty miserable affairs, mostly
because they involve not
eating. But quite frankly,
I'm too much of a food lover
to ever try anything quite
that extreme.

FOOD PLAN & RECIPES

And the good news is, you don't have to. While this 7-day cleanse will strip calories out of your day—reducing inflammation, bloating and fat storage along the way—I don't want you to go hungry. In fact, studies show that certain foods actually improve the effectiveness of the catechins found in tea. In particular, studies show that those who have low levels of serum albumin—a type of protein found in the blood—also have lower levels of catechins, the active compound in tea. Albumin is essential for moving fluids and nutrients between the bloodstream and the body tissues. Eating enough lean protein is the key to keeping those blood albumin levels up.

While I've included an array of great recipes for you to sample— both during your cleanse and in the weeks and months ahead—my goal is to make the next 7 days exceedingly simple. So rather than force you to follow recipes—easy as they may be—I've assembled instead a simple menu of proteins, vegetables and starches for you to choose from. Just pick one of each, and you've got a perfect Flat-Belly Tea Cleanse dinner!

PROTEIN CHOICES
CHOOSE ONE EACH NIGHT

FISH *5 oz fillet per person*
(will cook down to about 3-4 oz portion)

Wild Caught Alaskan Salmon

→ Lightly drizzle low sodium soy sauce and teriyaki sauce. Throw in fresh ginger, garlic, and pineapple for added nutrition

→ Bake at 400 degrees for about 15 minutes

200 calories, 21 g protein, 11 g fat

Wild Pacific/Alaskan Halibut

→ Brush with honey and Dijon mustard, squeeze lemon slices and leave them on top

→ Steam inside a sealed foil packet on baking pan in the oven at 400 degrees for 15 minutes or throw the foil packet on the grill until the internal temp reads 140–145 degrees

115 calories, 22 g protein, 2.5 g fat

Farmed Rainbow Trout

→ Brush with olive oil, rub with your favorite seasoning (Italian seasoning, Old Bay, etc) and a dash of salt and pepper, squeeze fresh lemon juice over top

→ Broil in preheated oven, 4–5 minutes each side

117 calories, 18 g protein, 4.6 g fat

CHICKEN

skinless breast halves, one half per person

170 calories, 25 g protein, 7 g fat per 3 oz cooked portion

Salsa Chicken

→ Place chicken in baking dish, pour your favorite salsa over, enough to cover the chicken

→ Throw in ½ cup black beans and ½ cup corn to increase nutrition

→ Bake at 375 degrees for 30-40 minutes

Marinated Chicken

→ Marinate chicken for 30-60 minutes in a vinaigrette such as balsamic, raspberry, etc

→ Sprinkle with fresh or dried herbs such as rosemary, thyme or minced garlic

→ Bake at 375 degrees for 30-40 minutes

EGGS

70 calories, 5 g fat, 6 g protein per egg

Dinner Frittata

→ Beat 2 eggs with 2 tbsp 2 percent milk, sprinkle of favorite dried herbs, salt, pepper

→ Add ½ cup favorite chopped veggies such as peppers, tomatoes, broccoli

→ Heat 2 tsp butter in small frying pan and pour in egg mixture, cook over low/medium about 8–10 minutes

Egg Wrap

→ Layer 2 poached or scrambled eggs, avocado slices, and fresh salsa on a wrap

→ Garnish with cilantro and Tabasco sauce to taste

FOOD PLAN & RECIPES

VEGETABLE CHOICES

BROCCOLI *steamed or roasted, one cup chopped*

31 calories, 2.4 g fiber

ASPARAGUS *steamed or roasted, one cup chopped*

27 calories, 2.8 g fiber

BELL PEPPERS *steamed or roasted, one cup chopped*

39 calories, 3.1 g fiber

RAW CHOPPED BABY KALE

17 calories, 1 g fiber, 1 g protein

RAW CHOPPED BABY SPINACH

10 calories, 1 g fiber, 1 g protein

BRUSSELS SPROUTS *cut in half and sautéed or roasted, one cup*

56 calories, 4.1 g fiber, 4 g protein

ZUCCHINI/YELLOW SUMMER SQUASH *sautéed or roasted, one cup chopped*

20 calories, 1 g fiber, 2 g protein

STARCH CHOICES

QUINOA *1 cup cooked*
222 calories, 4 g fat, 5 g fiber, 8 g protein

BROWN RICE *1 cup cooked*
216 calories, 1.8 g fat, 3.5 g fiber, 5 g protein

SWEET POTATO *one medium baked*
100 calories, 3.7 g fiber, 2.2 g protein

FARRO *1 cup cooked*
220 calories, 2 g fat, 5 g fiber, 8 g protein

BULGUR WHEAT *1 cup cooked*
151 calories, 0.4 g fat, 8 g fiber, 6 g protein

GARBANZO BEANS *½ cup cooked*
106 calories, 2.1 g fat, 5 g fiber, 5.4 g protein

EDAMAME *½ cup shelled and boiled*
127 calories, 5.8 g fat, 3.8 g fiber, 11.1 g protein

Simple enough, right? But if you want to delve deeper into the potential of your own kitchen, try whipping up one of these exciting recipes.

Black Bean Omelet

Why shell out your hard-earned dollars for an overpriced gut bomb when you can make something better, healthier, and cheaper at home in 10 minutes flat? That is the question that you face with many restaurant dishes, and nowhere is it more relevant than with omelets. Which would you prefer: an $11 spinach omelet with nearly 1,000 calories, or a $1.50 omelet filled with an oozing center of black beans and cheese, for 330 calories?

YOU'LL NEED

1   can (14–16 oz) black beans, drained

     Juice of 1 lime

¼ tsp cumin

     Hot sauce to taste

8   eggs

     Salt and black pepper to taste

½ cup feta cheese, plus more for serving

     Bottled salsa

     Sliced avocado (optional)

HOW TO MAKE IT

→ Pulse the black beans, lime juice, cumin, and a few shakes of hot sauce in a food processor until it has the consistency of refried beans, adding a bit of water to help if necessary.

→ Coat a small nonstick pan with nonstick cooking spray or a bit of butter or olive oil and heat over medium heat. Crack two eggs into a bowl and beat with a bit of salt and pepper. Add the eggs to the pan, then use a spatula to stir and then lift the cooked egg on the bottom to allow raw egg to slide under. When the eggs have all but set, spoon a quarter of the black bean mixture and 2 tablespoons feta down the middle of the omelet. Use the spatula to fold over a third of the egg to cover the mixture in the center, then carefully slide the omelet onto a plate, using the spatula flip it over at the last second to form one fully rolled omelet.

→ Repeat with the remaining ingredients to make four omelets. Garnish with salsa, avocado slices if you like, and a bit more crumbled feta.

MAKES 4 SERVINGS → COST PER SERVING: $1.47

330 calories, 8 g fat (6 g saturated), 480 mg sodium

Sesame Noodles with Chicken

Italians might cringe in horror to hear it, but the noodle originally comes from Asia. In 2005, archaeologists discovered what they believe to be the oldest bowl of noodles on record, dating back some 4,000 years. (No word yet on what type of sauce they were dressed with.) The point being that sometimes a box of fettuccine is just as appropriate for an Asian-inspired meal as it is for an Italian repast. Think of this as a salad, with the noodles sitting in for lettuce. Add some protein and as many or as few vegetables as you like, and toss the whole package with a light but powerful dressing. It's the culmination of four millennia of noodle knowledge. (Well, maybe not, but it's awfully tasty.)

YOU'LL NEED

- 6 oz whole-wheat fettuccine
- 2 tsp toasted sesame oil, plus more for noodles
- Juice of 1 lime
- 2 Tbsp warm water
- 1½ Tbsp chunky peanut butter
- 1½ Tbsp low-sodium soy sauce
- 2 tsp chili sauce, such as sriracha
- 2 cups shredded cooked chicken
- 1 red or yellow bell pepper, sliced
- 2 cups sugar snap peas
- 1 cup cooked and shelled edamame (optional)
- Chopped peanuts, sesame seeds, or chopped scallions (optional)

HOW TO MAKE IT

→ Bring a large pot of salted water to a boil and cook the pasta according to package instructions. Drain the pasta and toss in a large bowl with a bit of sesame oil to keep the noodles from sticking.

→ Combine the lime juice, water, peanut butter, soy sauce, chili sauce, and sesame oil in a microwave-safe mixing bowl. Microwave for 45 seconds, then stir to create a uniform sauce.

→ Add the sauce to the noodles and toss to mix. Stir in the chicken, bell pepper, sugar snaps, and edamame, if using. Top individual servings with peanuts, sesame seeds, or scallions if you like.

MAKES 4 SERVINGS → COST PER SERVING $2.05

340 calories, 11 g fat (2 g saturated), 400 mg sodium

FOOD PLAN & RECIPES

Grilled Vegetable Wrap

Can it be? A truly healthy wrap? I've been watching on the sidelines in shock and dismay as one person after the next is tricked into believing that a wrap is some sort of magical weight-loss bullet. Unfortunately, sandwich shops and sit-down spots alike take advantage of the reputation to cram Frisbee-size tortillas with cheese, bacon, ranch, and any other high-calorie ingredients they can find. Even with a dusting of goat cheese and a spread of balsamic mayo, this wrap earns its healthy stripes by virtue of its low calorie counts and generous vegetable filling.

YOU'LL NEED

- 12 asparagus spears, woody ends removed
- 2 portobello mushroom caps
- 1 red bell pepper, halved, seeds and stem removed
- 1 Tbsp olive oil

  Salt and black pepper to taste
- 2 Tbsp olive oil mayonnaise
- 1 Tbsp balsamic vinegar
- 1 clove garlic, minced
- 4 large spinach or whole-wheat tortillas or wraps
- 2 cups arugula, baby spinach, or mixed baby greens
- ¾ cup crumbled goat or feta cheese

THE 7-DAY FLAT-BELLY TEA CLEANSE

HOW TO MAKE IT

→ Preheat a grill. In a large bowl, toss the asparagus, mushrooms, and bell pepper with the olive oil, plus a few pinches of salt and pepper. Place the vegetables on the hottest part of the grill and cook, turning occasionally, until lightly charred and tender. The asparagus should take the least amount of time (about 5 minutes) and the peppers the most (about 10). (Alternatively, you can roast the vegetables in a 450°F oven for 10 to 12 minutes.) Slice the mushroom caps into thin strips. If possible, peel off the charred skin of the pepper and then slice.

→ Combine the mayonnaise, vinegar, and garlic and stir to combine thoroughly. Heat the tortillas on the grill or in the microwave for 30 seconds. Spread the balsamic mayo down the middle of each tortilla, then top with the greens and cheese. Divide the grilled vegetables among the tortillas, then roll up tightly and slice each wrap in half.

MAKES 4 SERVINGS → COST PER SERVING: $3.15

240 calories, 13 g fat (3.5 g saturated), 450 mg sodium

Avocado-Crab Salad

Crab doesn't come out much in the kitchen, but when it does, the idea is to do as little to it as possible. Otherwise, why spend the money on such a delicate ingredient? With the exception of a few salty Marylanders, nobody knows crabs better than the cooks of Southeast Asia, so this recipe follows their light-handed lead, incorporating cucumbers and onion for crunch, chilies for heat, and a bit of fish or soy sauce for a touch of savory salt. An avocado half makes the perfect vessel for this salad, its rich, creamy texture boosting the sweetness of the crab.

YOU'LL NEED

1	can (8 oz) crabmeat, preferably jumbo lump, drained
½	cup diced, seeded and peeled cucumber
¼	cup minced red onion
¼	cup chopped fresh cilantro
1	jalapeño pepper (preferably red), minced
1	Tbsp fish sauce (in a pinch, soy sauce will do)
1	Tbsp sugar
	Juice of 1 lime
	Salt
4	small Haas avocados, halved and pitted
1	lime, quartered

THE 7-DAY FLAT-BELLY TEA CLEANSE

HOW TO MAKE IT

→ Combine the crab, cucumber, onion, cilantro, jalapeño, fish
sauce, sugar, and lime juice in a mixing bowl. Stir gently to combine, being careful not to break up the bigger lumps of crab.
Lightly salt the flesh of the avocados, then divide the crab mixture
among the 8 halves, spooning it directly into the bowls created
by removing the pits. Serve with the lime quarters.

MAKES 4 SERVINGS → COST PER SERVING: $3.55

355 calories, 25 g fat (4 g saturated), 550 mg sodium

Chinese Chicken Salad

Chinese chicken salad is one of the world's ultimate fusion foods. It's an Eastern-inspired dish popularized by an Austrian chef (Wolfgang Puck) in Beverly Hills (at his restaurant Spago back in the 1980s). Whatever its disparate origins, it's undeniably one of the most popular—and ubiquitous—salads in America, sharing space on menus in four-star restaurants and Wendy's alike. Too bad most versions are nutritional disasters, bogged down by too much dressing and too many fried noodles. This lighter version is true to Wolfgang's original inspiration but with about a third of the calories.

YOU'LL NEED

1	head napa cabbage
½	head red cabbage
½	Tbsp sugar
2	cups chopped or shredded cooked chicken (freshly grilled or from a store-bought rotisserie chicken)
⅓	cup bottled Asian vinaigrette
1	cup fresh cilantro leaves
1	cup canned mandarin oranges, drained
¼	cup sliced almonds, toasted
	Salt and black pepper to taste

HOW TO MAKE IT

→ Slice the cabbages in half lengthwise and remove the cores. Slice the cabbage into thin strips. Toss with the sugar in a large bowl.

→ If the chicken is cold, toss with a few tablespoons of vinaigrette in a microwave-safe bowl and heat in a microwave at 50% power until warm. Add to the cabbage, along with the cilantro, mandarins, almonds, and the remaining vinaigrette. Toss to combine. Season with salt and pepper.

MAKES 4 SERVINGS → COST PER SERVING: $3.30

380 calories, 21 g fat (3.5 saturated), 23 g carbohydrates

Asian Beef Noodle Soup

When it comes to soups that serve as meals, no one can touch the Asian cuisines. From the thick, heady ramens of Japan to the funky, darkly satisfying beef noodle soups of China, to the spice-suffused bowls of pho from Vietnam, the entire continent seems to have mastered the art of transforming a few scraps of meat and vegetables into a magical eating experience. The slow-cooker soup here takes a cue from all three, combining a rich ginger- and soy-spiked broth with chunks of fork-tender beef, a tangle of springy noodles, and—for a fresh, high note to pair with the dark, brooding ones—a pile of fresh bok choy. This is no appetizer soup; this is a full-on meal.

YOU'LL NEED

- ½ Tbsp peanut or canola oil
- 1½ pounds chuck roast, cut into ½" chunks

  Salt and black pepper to taste
- 4 cups low-sodium beef broth
- 6 cups water
- ¼ cup low-sodium soy sauce
- 2 medium onions, roughly chopped
- 4 cloves garlic, peeled
- 1 piece fresh ginger (about 1-inch long), peeled and sliced into thin coins
- 4 whole star anise pods
- 12 oz Japanese udon noodles, rice noodles, or fettuccine
- 1 head bok choy, leaves chopped into 1" pieces, stems thinly sliced

  Fresh cilantro leaves and/or fresh basil leaves for garnish

  Sriracha and/or hoisin sauce for serving

HOW TO MAKE IT

→ Heat the oil in a large pot over high heat. Season the beef all over with salt and pepper. Working in batches if necessary, sear the beef on all sides for 3 to 4 minutes, until browned. Transfer to a slow cooker and add the broth, water, soy sauce, onions, garlic, ginger, and star anise. Cover and cook on low for 6 hours, until the beef is very tender. (Or simmer everything in the pot over a very low flame for 2 to 3 hours.)

→ When the beef is nearly ready, prepare the noodles according to package instructions. Add the bok choy to the soup and simmer for about 10 minutes, until tender. Season to taste with salt (if it needs any) and plenty of black pepper. Divide the noodles among 8 large bowls. Ladle the broth, along with a generous amount of beef and bok choy, into each bowl. Top with cilantro and basil (if using) and serve with sriracha and/or hoisin sauce.

MAKES 8 SERVINGS → COST PER SERVING: $2.44

350 calories, 8 g fat (2 g saturated), 550 mg sodium

Thai Beef Lettuce Wraps

Asian cultures have known for hundreds (if not thousands) of years that wrapping things in lettuce makes an amazing snack or meal. Too bad the restaurant industry got its claws on the idea and fiddled with its simple brilliance. Now wraps at places like P.F. Chang's and Cheesecake Factory are overwrought affairs packing as many calories into an appetizer as you should have in an entire meal. Consider this Vietnamese-inspired version a blissful, healthy, flavor-packed return to the wrap's humble roots.

YOU'LL NEED

12 oz flank, skirt, or sirloin steak

Salt and black pepper to taste

 1 Tbsp hot sauce (preferably sriracha)

 2 Tbsp fish sauce

Juice of 1 lime, plus wedges as garnish

 1 jalapeño pepper, thinly sliced

½ red onion, thinly sliced

½ cup chopped fresh cilantro

 1 carrot, grated

 1 head Bibb lettuce, leaves separated

HOW TO MAKE IT

→ Heat the grill to hot or heat a grill pan over high heat for at least 5 minutes. Season the steak with salt and pepper and toss it onto the grill. Cook for about 4 minutes on each side, until it's firm but yielding to the touch. Let it rest for 5 minutes.

→ Combine the hot sauce, fish sauce, and juice of 1 lime in a small saucepan over low heat.

→ Slice the steak thinly (if it's flank or skirt steak, be sure to cut across the grain) and drizzle half of the warm sauce over it. Set out the jalapeño and onion slices, cilantro, carrot, and lettuce, along with the lime wedges and sauce. Use the leaves like tortillas to wrap up the steak slices with the other ingredients.

MAKES 2 SERVINGS → COST PER SERVING: $4.86

290 calories, 8 g fat (3 g saturated), 1,020 mg sodium

Zucchini Carbonara

Spaghetti carbonara is the Italians' take on bacon and eggs. It's comfort food at its finest: simple, unpretentious, soul nourishing. The only problem is that a pile of bacon-strewn pasta won't win any nutrition awards. Combine that with the fact that most American restaurants add heavy cream to carbonara—a huge no-no in Italy—and things get even worse. To lighten the dish, we've added a good amount of zucchini, which is cut in long, thin ribbons to mimic the shape of the pasta and help you cut back on the overall quantity of noodles. Beyond cutting calories, though, it adds a nutty sweetness to this classic that just makes a lot of sense. (Just don't tell the Italians, okay?)

YOU'LL NEED

- 10 oz spaghetti
- 6 strips bacon, cut into ½" pieces
- 1 medium yellow onion, diced
- 1 large zucchini, sliced into thin ribbons
- 2 cloves garlic, sliced
  Salt and black pepper to taste
- 2 eggs
  Pecorino or Parmesan for grating
- 1 handful chopped fresh parsley

HOW TO MAKE IT

→ Bring a large pot of salted water to a boil. Add the pasta and cook until al dente (usually about 30 seconds to a minute less than the package instructions recommend).

→ While the pasta cooks, heat a large sauté pan over medium heat. Add the bacon and cook until crispy, about 5 minutes. Transfer the bacon to a plate lined with paper towels. Discard all but a thin film of the fat from the pan. Add the onion, zucchini, and garlic and cook for 5 to 7 minutes, until soft and lightly browned. Stir back in the bacon and season with a bit of salt and plenty of coarse black pepper.

→ Drain the pasta, using a coffee cup to save a few ounces of the cooking water. Add the pasta directly to the sauté pan and toss to coat. Stir in enough of the pasta water so that a thin layer of moisture clings to the noodles. Remove from the heat and crack the two eggs directly into the pasta, using tongs or two forks to toss for even distribution. Divide the pasta among four warm bowls or plates and top with grated cheese and parsley.

MAKES 4 SERVINGS → COST PER SERVING: $1.72

370 calories, 8 g fat (3 g saturated), 960 mg sodium

Honey-Mustard Salmon

Many Americans view fresh fish as restaurant fare, food best left to professionals to skillfully prepare. But when you leave the fish cooking to "professionals" at places like Outback, Friday's, and Applebee's, your hopes of a healthy dinner may be sunk. Why blow the cash and the heavy caloric toll on a meal you can prepare at home in less time than it takes to order out? Plus, if you ever hope to get a kid to eat fish, this 3-minute sauce (which goes great on shrimp, scallops, and chicken, as well) is the key.

YOU'LL NEED

- 1 Tbsp butter
- 1 Tbsp brown sugar
- 2 Tbsp Dijon mustard
- 1 Tbsp honey
- 1 Tbsp soy sauce
- ½ Tbsp olive oil

  Salt and black pepper to taste
- 4 salmon fillets (6 oz each)

HOW TO MAKE IT

→ Preheat the oven to 400°F. Combine the butter and brown sugar in a bowl and microwave for 30 seconds, until the butter and sugar have melted together. Stir in the mustard, honey, and soy sauce.

→ Heat the oil in an ovenproof skillet over high heat. Season the salmon with salt and pepper and add to the pan flesh side down. Cook for 3 to 4 minutes until fully browned and flip. Brush with half of the glaze and place the pan in the oven until the salmon is firm and flaky (but before the white fat begins to form on the surface), about 5 minutes. Remove, brush the salmon with more of the honey mustard.

MAKES 4 SERVINGS → COST PER SERVING: $2.77

370 calories, 21 g fat (6 g saturated), 530 mg sodium

FOOD PLAN & RECIPES

Halibut in a Bag

A hunk of halibut is one of the planet's healthiest foods. A hunk of halibut smothered in butter and half a day's worth of sodium is decidedly not. This recipe uses a simple—but often overlooked—technique and a handful of potent flavor builders to create one of the most perfectly balanced meals in this entire book.

YOU'LL NEED

- 2 fillets of halibut or other firm white fish (5 oz each)
- 1 jar (8 oz) marinated artichoke hearts, drained
- 1 cup cherry tomatoes
- 2 Tbsp chopped kalamata olives
- ½ medium fennel bulb, thinly sliced
- 1 lemon, half cut into thin slices, the other half cut into quarters
- ½ Tbsp olive oil
- ¼ cup dry white wine

  Salt and black pepper to taste

HOW TO MAKE IT

→ Preheat the oven to 400°F.

→ Take 2 large sheets of parchment paper or foil, place a fillet in the center of each, and top equally with the artichokes, tomatoes, olives, fennel, and lemon slices. Drizzle with the olive oil and wine; season with salt and pepper. Fold the paper or foil over the fish and seal by tightly rolling up the edges, creating a secure pouch. It's important the packets are fully sealed so that the steam created inside can't escape.

→ Place the pouches on a baking sheet in the center of the oven and bake for 20 to 25 minutes, depending on how thick the fish is. Serve with the remaining lemon wedges.

MAKES 2 SERVINGS → COST PER SERVING: $9.50

300 calories, 8 g fat (1 g saturated), 870 mg sodium

Summer Roll with Shrimp and Mango

Not to be confused with the deep-fried spring roll, the summer roll is a prime example of how a few healthy, relatively boring ingredients can be carefully coerced into something much greater than the sum of their parts. The combination of shrimp, sweet mango, and crunchy strips of red pepper makes for seriously good eating, but once you master the simple wrapping technique, feel free to fiddle with the filling.

YOU'LL NEED

- 1 Tbsp chunky peanut butter
- 1 Tbsp sugar
- ½ Tbsp fish sauce
- ½ Tbsp rice wine vinegar, plus more for the noodles
- 2 oz vermicelli or thin rice noodles (capellini or angel hair pasta also works)
- 8 sheets of rice paper
- ½ lb cooked medium shrimp, each sliced in half
- ½ red bell pepper, thinly sliced
- 1 mango, peeled, pitted, and cut into thin strips
- 4 scallion greens, cut into thin strips
- ¼ cup cilantro or mint leaves

HOW TO MAKE IT

→ Combine the peanut butter, sugar, fish sauce, and vinegar with 1 tablespoon warm water. Stir to thoroughly combine. Set the peanut sauce aside.

→ Cook the noodles according to package instructions. Drain and toss with a few shakes of vinegar to keep them from sticking.

→ Dip a sheet of rice paper in a bowl of warm water for a few seconds, until just soft and bendable. Lay the paper on a cutting board. Leaving a ½" space at each end of the wrapper, top with noodles, 3 or 4 shrimp halves, bell pepper, mango, scallion, and a few whole cilantro leaves. Fold the ends of the rice paper toward the center, then roll tight like a burrito. Repeat with the remaining 7 wrappers. Serve with the peanut sauce.

MAKES 4 SERVINGS → COST PER SERVING: $3.02

270 calories, 3.5 g fat (0 g saturated), 390 mg sodium

Seared Ahi with Ginger-Scallion Sauce

As much as I love ahi tuna for its profusion of lean protein and heart-strengthening, brain-boosting omega-3 fatty acids, what I love most about the fish is the fact that even a kitchen neophyte can cook it perfectly in less than 5 minutes. All it takes is a pan set over high heat, a touch of oil, and a sprinkle of salt and pepper. I add bok choy to make this a more nutritious, substantial dish, but any green vegetable (spinach, broccoli, asparagus) will do. Just don't skip the ginger-scallion sauce, a ubiquitous Chinatown condiment good enough to make a pair of old socks into a memorable meal.

YOU'LL NEED

1	bunch scallions, bottoms removed, finely chopped
2	Tbsp fresh ginger, peeled and grated
1	Tbsp low-sodium soy sauce
3	Tbsp peanut oil
1	Tbsp rice wine vinegar
16	oz ahi or other high-quality tuna steaks
	Salt and pepper to taste
½	lb shiitake mushrooms, stems removed, sliced
1	lb baby bok choy, stems removed

HOW TO MAKE IT

→ Combine the scallions, ginger, soy sauce, 2 tablespoons of the oil, and vinegar in a mixing bowl and stir thoroughly to combine. Set aside. (Making this ahead and storing in the refrigerator is not only possible but advisable, as even 30 minutes of sitting allows the flavors to marry nicely.)

→ Heat the remaining oil in a large cast-iron skillet or sauté pan. Season the tuna liberally with salt and lots of black pepper. When the oil is lightly smoking, add the tuna to the pan and sear for 2 minutes on each side, until deeply browned. Remove.

→ While the tuna rests, add the shiitake mushrooms to the same hot pan. (Use another drizzle of oil if the pan is dry.) Cook for 2 to 3 minutes, until lightly browned, then add the bok choy. Cook for another 2 to 3 minutes, until the bok choy is lightly wilted. Season to taste with salt and pepper.

→ Slice the tuna into thick strips. Divide the bok choy and mushrooms among 4 warm plates. Top with slices of tuna, then drizzle with the ginger-scallion sauce.

MAKES 4 SERVINGS → COST PER SERVING: $5.38

301 calories, 12 g fat (2 g saturated), 271 mg sodium

Thai Chicken Curry

Redolent of ginger and lemongrass, chilies and coconut milk, Thai curry brings all of the classic flavors of Southeast Asian cuisine—salty, sour, bitter, hot—together in one dish. What's more, it derives its flavor from ingredients packed with powerful antioxidants. Even coconut milk contains lauric acid, among the healthiest forms of fat you can consume. The flavors may be exotic, but the tender chicken, the bouquet of vegetables, and the rich coconut milk will all taste wonderfully familiar.

YOU'LL NEED

1   Tbsp peanut or canola oil

1   large onion, sliced

2   cloves garlic, minced

2   tsp minced fresh ginger

1   Tbsp red curry paste

1   can (14 oz) light coconut milk

1   cup chicken broth

1   large sweet potato, peeled and cut into cubes

8   oz green beans

1   lb boneless, skinless chicken breasts, sliced into ¼"-thick pieces

   Juice of 1 lime

1   Tbsp fish sauce (optional)

   Chopped fresh cilantro or basil, for garnish

   Steamed brown rice

HOW TO MAKE IT

→ Heat the oil in a large saucepan or pot over medium heat. Add the onions, garlic, and ginger and sauté for about 5 minutes, until soft and fragrant. Add the curry paste, cook for a few minutes, then stir in the coconut milk and broth and bring to a simmer.

→ Add the sweet potato and simmer for 10 minutes. Stir in the green beans and chicken and cook for about 5 minutes, until the vegetables are just tender and the chicken is cooked through. Stir in the lime juice and fish sauce, if using. Serve over steamed brown rice, garnished with cilantro or basil, if you like.

MAKES 4 SERVINGS → COST PER SERVING $3.17

340 calories, 13 g fat (6 g saturated), 400 mg sodium

Asian Tuna Burgers with Wasabi Mayo

A firm, meaty fish like tuna is prime picking for the burger treatment. All it takes is a quick pulse in the food processor, or even just a bit of fine chopping. Either way, make sure the fish is very cold, which keeps the proteins from binding into tough lumps. The resulting ground tuna is ready to be formed into patties and dressed up in dozens of different ways. If tuna isn't your fish of choice, salmon works every bit as well.

YOU'LL NEED

- 1 lb fresh tuna
- 4 scallions, minced
- 1 tsp minced fresh ginger
- 1 Tbsp low-sodium soy sauce
- 1 tsp toasted sesame oil
-    Canola oil, for grilling
- 2 Tbsp olive oil mayonnaise
- ½ Tbsp prepared wasabi (from powder or in premade paste)
- 4 whole-wheat sesame buns, split and lightly toasted
- 1 cup sliced cucumber, lightly salted
- 2 cups mixed baby greens

HOW TO MAKE IT

→ Chop the tuna into ½" cubes, then place in the freezer for 10 minutes to firm up. (This will make grinding easier.) Working in batches if necessary, pulse the tuna in a food processor to the consistency of ground beef. (Be sure not to overdo it; you only want to pulse it only enough so that you can form patties.) Transfer to a mixing bowl and mix in the scallions, ginger, soy sauce, and sesame oil. Form into 4 equal patties. Place in the fridge for at least 10 minutes before grilling to firm up.

→ Preheat a well-oiled grill or grill pan. When hot, add the patties and cook for 2 to 3 minutes each side, until browned on the outside, but still medium rare in the center. Flip and handle carefully, as these burgers are more delicate than beef burgers.

→ Mix the mayo with the wasabi in a small bowl, then spread evenly onto the bun tops. Line the bottoms with cucumber and greens, top with the burgers, then crown with the bun tops.

MAKES 4 SERVINGS → COST PER SERVING: $3.82

330 calories, 11 g fat (2 g saturated), 460 mg sodium

Tortilla Soup

Over the past two decades, tortilla soup has rivaled chicken soup as a comforting mainstay on major restaurant menus. Between the pulled chicken, the soothing tomato broth, and the pile of fixings, what's not to love? How about a bowl of soup with 86 percent of your day's sodium allotment? Unless you learn to enjoy it at home, that's what you're likely to get.

YOU'LL NEED

- 1 Tbsp canola oil
- 1 onion, chopped
- 2 cloves garlic, chopped
- 1 can (14 oz) whole peeled tomatoes
- 1 Tbsp chipotle pepper
- 6 cups chicken broth
- ¾ lb boneless, skinless chicken breasts

   Salt and black pepper to taste
- 2 corn tortillas, cut into strips

   Juice of 2 limes

   Hot sauce (optional)
- ½ avocado, pitted, peeled, and cut into cubes

   Chopped onion, pickled jalapeños, sliced radishes, fresh cilantro (optional)

THE 7-DAY FLAT-BELLY TEA CLEANSE

HOW TO MAKE IT

→ Heat the oil in a large pot over medium heat. Cook the onion and garlic until soft and translucent. Transfer to a blender and add the tomatoes (with juice) and chipotle; puree until smooth.

→ Return to the pot and add the broth. Bring to a simmer. Season the chicken with salt and pepper. Drop the breasts into the liquid whole. Poach them in the soup until cooked all the way through, about 10 minutes. Remove and slice thin just before serving.

→ Preheat the oven to 450°F. Lay the tortilla strips on a baking sheet and bake until lightly brown and crispy.

→ Season the soup with the lime juice; adjust the seasoning with salt, pepper, and hot sauce (if using). Divide among 4 warm bowls. Top with the chicken, tortilla strips, avocado, and as many of the other garnishes as you'd like to use.

MAKES 4 SERVINGS → COST PER SERVING: $2.77

300 calories, 11 g fat (1.5 g saturated), 550 mg sodium

Sea Bass Packet

Why more people don't cook food in packets is one of the culinary world's great mysteries. Not only is it one of the healthiest, easiest ways to cook fish, chicken, and vegetables, but the abundance of flavorful steam trapped inside the packet means your food will still be delicious, even if you overcook it. Plus, there are no pots or pans to clean—just toss the foil in the trash and move on. Sure beats driving to a restaurant, waiting for a table, shelling out $22 for a 600-calorie piece of fish with more than a day's worth of sodium, and then driving home disappointed.

YOU'LL NEED

- 4   sea bass, halibut, or other white fish fillets (6 oz each)
- 8   spears asparagus, woody ends removed, chopped
- 4   oz shiitake mushrooms, stems removed
- 1   Tbsp grated fresh ginger
- 2   Tbsp low-sodium soy sauce
- 2   Tbsp mirin (sweetened sake), sake, or sweet white wine

    Salt and black pepper to taste

HOW TO MAKE IT

→ Preheat the oven to 400°F.

→ Lay 4 large (18-by-12-inch) pieces of aluminum foil on the kitchen counter and fold each into thirds. Place a fish fillet in the center third of each piece, then scatter the asparagus, mushrooms, and ginger over each. Drizzle with the soy sauce and mirin and season with a small pinch of salt (remember, soy sauce already packs plenty of sodium) and black pepper. Fold the outer two sections of the foil over the fish, then roll up the ends toward the center to create fully sealed packets.

→ Arrange the packets on a large baking sheet and bake for 15 for 20 minutes, depending on the thickness of the fish fillets. (If the fillets are ½-inch thick or less, they will take closer to 15 minutes to bake; if they are almost a full inch, they will need 20 minutes.) Place each packet directly on a plate and serve.

MAKES 4 SERVINGS → COST PER SERVING: $5.85

250 calories, 4.5 g fat (1 g saturated), 540 mg sodium

Pesto-Grilled Swordfish

No fridge should be without a bottle of premade pesto. It pairs perfectly with pasta, of course, but also works as an excellent sandwich spread, salad dressing enhancer, and instant marinade. This recipe takes the latter tack, slathering meaty swordfish steaks in pesto before grilling, then topping them with quick-sautéed tomatoes. The burst of sweetness from the tomatoes joins forces with the garlicky punch of the pesto, making for a dish that tastes every bit the creation of a restaurant chef.

YOU'LL NEED

- 2 Tbsp bottled pesto
- 4 swordfish steaks (4–6 oz each)
- 1 Tbsp olive oil
- 2 cloves garlic, peeled and lightly crushed
- 2 cups cherry tomatoes
-   Salt and black pepper to taste

HOW TO MAKE IT

→ Spread the pesto all over the swordfish steaks, cover, and marinate in the fridge for 30 minutes.

→ While the fish marinates, heat the olive oil in a sauté pan over medium heat. Add the garlic and cook for 1 to 2 minutes, until lightly browned. Add the tomatoes and sauté until the skins are lightly blistered and about to pop, about 5 minutes. Season with salt and pepper.

→ Preheat a grill or grill pan. Season the fish all over with salt and pepper. When the grill is hot, cook the swordfish for 4 to 5 minutes per side, until the fish is cooked all the way through and the flesh flakes with gentle pressure. Reheat the tomatoes and top each steak with a scoop.

MAKES 4 SERVINGS → COST PER SERVING: $5.05

250 calories, 13 g fat (3 g saturated), 390 mg sodium

Spicy Thai Chicken with Basil

The cuisines of Southeast Asia—Thai, Vietnamese, Malaysian—deliver more flavor per calorie than any other on the planet and make for a refreshing break from the cartons of Chinese takeout that clutter so many American refrigerators. This Thai classic (called gai pad grapow) gets its flavor from chilies, garlic, and fresh herbs—nutritional powerhouses known to boost metabolism and fight cancer. Together, they also make for a full-throttle flavor experience that trumps nearly any Chinese stir-fry in the health department. Adjust the heat to your liking, but if it's not at least somewhat fiery, then it's not Thai.

YOU'LL NEED

- 1   Tbsp peanut or canola oil
- 1   medium red onion, thinly sliced
- 2   jalapeño peppers, thinly sliced (or more if you really like your food fiery)
- 4   cloves garlic, minced
- 1   lb boneless, skinless chicken breasts, cut into small pieces
- 2   Tbsp fish sauce
- 1   Tbsp sugar
- 1   Tbsp low-sodium soy sauce
- 2   cups fresh basil leaves (preferably Thai or holy basil, but you'll find those only at specialty markets)

    Brown rice

THE 7-DAY FLAT-BELLY TEA CLEANSE

HOW TO MAKE IT

→ Heat the oil in a wok or large skillet. When hot, add the onion, jalapeños, and garlic and stir-fry for 2 minutes, using a metal spatula to keep the ingredients in motion. Add the chicken and cook for 2 to 3 minutes, until the meat is beginning to brown on the outside. Add the fish sauce, sugar, soy sauce, and basil and cook for 1 minute more. Serve over brown rice.

MAKES 4 SERVINGS → COST PER SERVING: $1.67

190 calories, 6 g fat (1.5 g saturated), 890 mg sodium

Chicken with Tomato, Olives and Capers

Ever wonder why everything "tastes like chicken"? Because chicken doesn't taste like much in particular, making it a catchall canvas for describing other things that don't taste like anything. The good news is this chicken does taste like something: Roasting it with tomatoes, capers, and olive oil bastes the chicken in a savory broth, keeping the meat moist and ultimately providing both a chunky, textured topping and an intensely satisfying sauce to dump over the top. You can pull this off in a single baking dish, but the foil is there to catch all the drippings—and spare you the post-dinner cleanup.

YOU'LL NEED

4	boneless, skinless chicken breasts (4–6 oz each), pounded to uniform ¼" thickness
	Salt and black pepper to taste
1	pint cherry tomatoes or 2 cups chopped tomatoes
½	red onion, diced
¼	cup green olives, pitted and chopped
¼	cup pine nuts
2	Tbsp capers
2	Tbsp olive oil
	Thinly sliced fresh basil (optional)

THE 7-DAY FLAT-BELLY TEA CLEANSE

HOW TO MAKE IT

→ Preheat the oven to 450°F. Season the chicken with salt and pepper. Take 4 large sheets of aluminum foil and fold each in half, then fold up about 1" of each side to create 4 trays, each large enough to comfortably hold a chicken breast. Place a breast on each piece of foil.

→ Combine the tomatoes, onion, olives, pine nuts, capers, and olive oil with a few pinches of salt and pepper in a mixing bowl. Top the chicken breasts with the mixture.

→ Place the chicken trays on a baking sheet and bake for about 15 minutes, until the chicken is cooked through. Serve with the tomato mixture and any accumulated juices from the foil drizzled on top. Garnish with basil (if using).

MAKES 4 SERVINGS → COST PER SERVING: $2.93

310 calories, 18 g fat (2.5 g saturated), 420 mg sodium

Provençal Chicken

This is the type of simple, healthy, satisfying dish that gives Mediterranean cooking its reputation as the perfect fusion of flavor and nutrition. All of the key components—white wine, tomatoes, olives, herbs—have the distinct advantage of being both intensely flavorful and incredibly good for you. Truth be told, who knows if people in Provence eat their chicken like this, but it has the soul of southern France in every bite.

YOU'LL NEED

- 1 Tbsp olive oil
- 8 boneless, skinless chicken thighs (about 1½ lb total)

Salt and black pepper to taste

- 1 small yellow onion, minced
- 3 cloves garlic, minced
- 3 Roma tomatoes, diced
- 1 cup dry white wine
- 1 cup chicken broth
- 1 tsp herbes de Provence
- ¼ cup pitted kalamata olives, roughly chopped

Fresh basil for garnish (optional)

HOW TO MAKE IT

→ Heat the olive oil in a large sauté pan over medium-high heat. Season the chicken all over with salt and black pepper. Add the chicken to the pan and cook, turning once, for about 6 minutes total, until seared and nicely browned. (Work in 2 batches if need be, so as not to overcrowd the pan.) Remove the chicken to a plate and reserve.

→ To the same pan, add the onions, garlic, and tomatoes and cook for about 5 minutes, until the onions and tomatoes are very soft. Add the wine, broth, and herbes de Provence and bring the mixture to a simmer. Return the chicken to the pan and simmer uncovered, turning the chicken halfway through, for about 20 minutes, until the meat is very tender. Stir in the olives, garnish with basil if you like, and serve.

MAKES 4 SERVINGS → COST PER SERVING $2.77

340 calories, 15 g fat (2.5 g saturated), 680 mg sodium

Hoisin–Lime Duck Breasts

For most people, duck is restaurant food, only to be enjoyed at white-linen fine-dining palaces or out-of-the-way Chinese spots. That's unfortunate, since it's not only intensely enjoyable, but also surprisingly lean and prime for the open flame. Its rich flavor is best when tempered with sweetness and acidity, both of which you'll find in this Asian-inspired glaze. Be sure to score the duck, as it will allow the fat underneath the skin to render out, leaving you with a crispy crust and soft, supple meat.

YOU'LL NEED

- ¼   cup hoisin sauce
-      Juice of 2 limes
- 1   Tbsp low-sodium soy sauce
- 1   tsp toasted sesame oil
- 4   duck breasts (about 5 oz each)
-      Black pepper to taste

HOW TO MAKE IT

→ Preheat a grill or grill pan over medium heat. Combine the hoisin, lime juice, soy sauce, and sesame oil in a mixing bowl. Set aside half the sauce for serving.

→ Score the duck: Make 3 diagonal cuts through the skin, then rotate 90 degrees and make 3 more cuts, creating diamonds in the skin. Season with pepper.

→ Grill the breasts, skin side down, for 5 minutes, until the fat begins to render and a crust forms. Flip and baste with the hoisin mixture. Continue cooking and basting for 3 to 5 minutes, until the duck is firm but gently yielding to the touch and an instant-read thermometer inserted into the thickest part of the duck reads 135°F. Let the duck rest for 5 minutes before slicing. Serve with the reserved sauce.

MAKES 4 SERVINGS → COST PER SERVING: $2.65

230 calories, 8 g fat (2 g saturated), 470 mg sodium

Herb–Roasted Turkey Breast

A recent study from the Harvard School of Public Health found that consuming processed meats—high in sodium and chemical preservatives—every day could boost your risk of heart disease by up to 42 percent. This turkey breast is not only low in sodium and nitrate-free, but it also makes the most delicious turkey sandwiches you've ever tasted.

YOU'LL NEED

8	cups water
¾	cup salt
1	cup sugar
1	large boneless, skinless turkey breast (about 3 pounds)
2	cloves garlic, peeled
	Salt and black pepper to taste
1	Tbsp olive oil
½	Tbsp minced fresh rosemary

HOW TO MAKE IT

→ Combine the water, salt, and sugar in a pot large enough to hold the turkey and bring to a boil. Stir until the sugar and salt have fully dissolved. Remove from the heat and let cool to room temperature. Add the turkey breast, cover, and place in the fridge to brine for at least 4 hours and up to overnight.

→ Preheat the oven to 425°F. Remove the turkey from the brine, pat dry, and roll up into a tight log. Use butcher twine to tie 3 separate knots, about 2" apart, that will hold the turkey in this tight shape.

→ Finely mince the garlic, using a pinch of salt and the back of your knife to mash it into a paste. Combine with the olive oil and rosemary, then rub all over the turkey, along with a good amount of black pepper. Place the turkey in a large roasting pan and roast until a thermometer inserted into the center of the meat reads 160°F, about 1 hour. Let the turkey rest before slicing.

→ The turkey can be served as is with traditional sides, or will keep up to a week in the fridge for sandwiches.

MAKES 12 SERVINGS → **COST PER SERVING: $1.27**

140 calories, 2 g fat (0 g saturated), 520 mg sodium

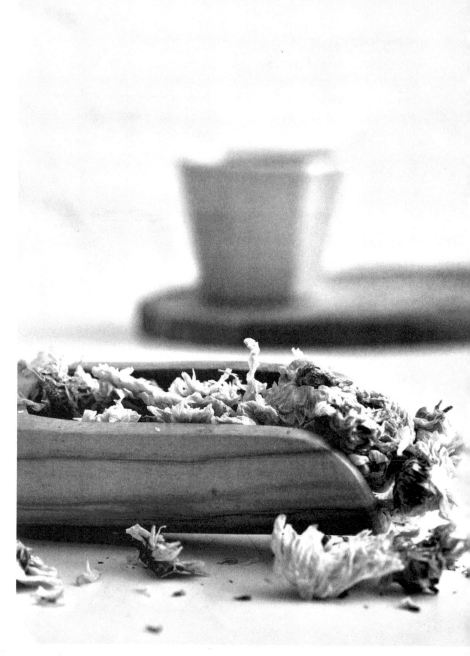

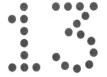

The Tea Cleanse Guide to Herbal Healing

For what ails you, from arthritis to headaches to the common cold. There's a drug-free remedy

Live longer, naturally, with no side effects. That's been the irresistible sales pitch for herbal remedies since plants first grew on Earth.

GUIDE TO HERBAL HEALING

So why are you hearing so much about them now, in this advanced new millennium? Because they'll also save you cash—an insane amount of cash, especially on drugs.

Americans spend more per capita on medicines than any other developed country, and buy more generics, too—and even the generics can cost $80 and up, since prices rose 5.3% in 2012. As a result, the natural-foods aisle is suddenly flooded with people trying to tell their cramp root from their dong quai. Vulnerable, hurting for money, we want to believe these cheaper remedies work. And do they?

This chapter tells you, definitively, which ones do—and which ones don't. I've combed through the most up-to-date research on botanical medicines, studying the latest breakthroughs and debunking the false claims. And I'm proud to report that relief is here for cancer, diabetes, even jet lag.

The idea behind herbal remedies is wonderfully simple: Herbalists believe whole plants are more effective than the isolated elements and synthetic ingredients used in drugs—with the added bonus of fewer unintentional effects. Herbal medicines should be seriously considered for ailments like colds and flu, insomnia, autoimmune diseases—the worries that typically cause conventional docs to throw up their hands. Yet herbs are also proven to help ease the symptoms of more serious ailments, like heart disease and cancer.

Chinese, Egyptian, Indian, and indigenous American civilizations might say, "Welcome to the club, America, what took you so long?" If trends here continue, it won't be long before this "boom" becomes common practice. While still not fully accepted by Western medicine or every M.D., herbal medicine is now taught more in medical and pharmacy schools. Extensive studies are ongoing not just overseas but now in the United States. And because some medical doctors realize that plants are the source of many synthetic drugs, an increasing number accept that herbs have benefit.

Just how much benefit? In this chapter, I recommend only products that fared well in evidence-based or double-blind studies—giving

THE 7-DAY FLAT-BELLY TEA CLEANSE

an honest look at what to buy and what to avoid. You'll find an A-to-Z Guide to Herbal Healing, the 9 best herbs for women, and sections on plants that can boost your mood, your energy, and your sex drive. As a sales pitch, it's irresistible; as medicine, it's sound.

What to Know Before You Buy

So, how safe are these products? And do they do what they promise? Well... it's tricky. Manufacturers do not need FDA approval to put their products on the market, and are allowed to put claims on the label, as long as they also note that the FDA hasn't approved the claim.

Once a product is on the market, the FDA does monitor its quality and safety, and if it's deemed unsafe, it can issue a warning or require the maker or distributor to remove the product from the marketplace. (In Europe and Australia, herbal products must provide scientific proof before any medicinal claims can be printed on labels.)

These guidelines do not, however, guarantee that an herb is safe for anyone to take—there may be dangerous interactions with other herbs or drugs, so always tell your medical doctor, and the herbal dispensary, about any drugs or herbal supplements you're on. Also:

Do your own research. This book offers a ton of research already and provides current warnings and precautions, but it's always a good idea to do some of your own and find out what support groups, studies and experts say about a particular herb.

Be especially careful if you are taking warfarin, aspirin, or any other blood-thinner; some herbs may increase their anticoagulant effect and increase the risk of bleeding. Some of these herbs are very innocent sounding, like chamomile and ginger. Also be careful if you are taking any immunosuppressant drugs—drugs that are used to suppress the immune system after a transplant or to control symptoms of autoimmune disease such as lupus and type-1 diabetes—such as corticosteroids (prednisone). Herbs that boost immunity, such as licorice, astragalus, and ginseng, may counteract these drugs.

Look for reputable brands. Many good companies are represented in these pages; try to buy from companies that have been in business for a long time and have an established reputation.

Learn how to read labels. A reputable brand will not just tell you its product will cure your headache—it should also tell you how, and you should be able to find ingredient descriptions and actions on the product website. Then you can cross-reference with unbiased, evidence-based research.

Follow label instructions. Duh. Don't think that if a little works well, a lot will work better. Just don't do it. And don't mix one herb with another herb, unless a professional tells you to.

Be smart. If you're pregnant or nursing, or have severe allergies or ailments, then don't take herbs without talking to your doctor. Don't give to children without talking to your doctor.

Tell your medical doctor what you're up to.
Unfortunately, a *New England Journal of Medicine* study found that 70% of people (mostly well-educated and with a high income) do not tell their doctors that they are using complementary or alternative treatments.

Healing Herbs A-to-Z

This is it: The List. The 23 herbs that have been proven to work—with a few bliss boosters and serenity savers as a bonus. Stick to the dosages specified here, in the studies, or on the label—and make sure to tell your doctor about any herbs you plan to take, especially if you are pregnant or nursing, have a chronic condition, or take medication regularly; remember that even though herbs are natural, they can still be contraindicated.

1 ALOE VERA
(Aloe barbadensis)

BEST FOR → **Burns**

Aloe vera is the herb for minor (second-degree) burns, confirmed by a 2009 *Surgery Today* study, among others that have shown aloe vera gel has a dramatic effect on burns, wounds and other skin conditions. The gel provides a protective layer for the affected area, and speeds healing due to aloecin B, which stimulates the immune system. The gel also can be used orally for ulcers and irritable bowel syndrome and as a laxative; it creates an internal protective coating and also stimulates the digestion.

DOSAGE: Apply 100% pure gel to burns several times a day—or, better yet, keep a potted plant on your windowsill and snip off a thick leaf, slit it open, and apply the gel to the burn. For ulcers, drink 50 milliliters a day.

PRECAUTIONS: Do not use the yellow gel at the base on skin. Do not take internally while pregnant or nursing or if suffering from kidney disease or hemorrhoids.

2 BOSWELLIA
(Boswellia serrata)

BEST FOR → Arthritis and joint injuries

Also known as Indian frankincense, this gummy resin has been clinically proven to have strong anti-inflammatory effects. Boswellia is known to reduce congestion and heat (kapha and pitta elements in ayurveda) in the joints, and is also used to promote appetite and digestion.

In a 2008 study published in *Arthritis Research & Therapy*, researchers gave people with osteoarthritis of the knee an extract of boswellia (5-Loxin). After three months, the herb group showed significantly greater relief than a group given a placebo.

DOSAGE: Take one 300-milligram capsule three times a day, with food.

3 ECHINACEA
(Echinacea angustifolia)

BEST FOR → Common cold

Studies on the effectiveness of echinacea for treating the common cold have been mixed. The largest so far was in 2012 at Cardiff University Common Cold Centre in the U.K., which found that three doses daily, taken for four months reduced the number of colds, and reduced the duration by 26%. The study was peer-reviewed and published in the journal *Evidence-Based Complementary and Alternative Medicine*. The study was funded by the Swiss manufacturers of Echinaforce. But many experts advise ignoring the naysayers, and following traditional usage.

"Native Americans used *Echinacea angustifolia*—not *Echinacea purpurea*—and they used only the root," explains Sheila Kingsbury, N.D., chair of the Department of Botanical Medicine at Bastyr University in Seattle. "Clinically speaking, accessing the root is the best place to start. It can shorten the length of a cold significantly."

DOSAGE: One teaspoon of echinacea root glycerite liquid every two hours beginning at onset of symptoms; decrease the dose to once every three to four hours after symptoms ease.

4 EVENING PRIMROSE OIL
(Oenothera)

BEST FOR → Eczema

Evening primrose seeds contain an oil with a high concentration of compounds rarely found in plants: the essential fatty acid gamma linolenic acid. There are more than 30 human studies reporting its benefits; in one, 1,207 patients found that the oil helped relieve the itching, swelling, crusting, and redness of eczema, which a 2013 University of Maryland Medical Center review confirms. It also has been found to lower blood pressure and reduce PMS and some multiple sclerosis symptoms when taken internally.

DOSAGE: Apply topically for skin conditions; follow label instructions for internal use.

5 FENNEL
(Foeniculum vulgare)

BEST FOR → Intestinal gas

Fennel seeds contain phytonutrients that are thought to reduce spasms in small muscle fibers like those found in the intestines, helping to reduce gassiness. The aromatic quality of the seeds will also help freshen your breath. And a 2011 review published in *Pediatrics*, for instance, found that fennel tea can be useful for treating a baby's gas-caused colic.

DOSAGE: Chew a pinch of whole fennel seeds after a meal. Your body will let you know—with one last burst of gas—when to stop.

6 FLAXSEED

(Linum usitatissimum)

BEST FOR → Heart health

Nearly twice as many American women die of heart disease and stroke as from all forms of cancer, including breast cancer, according to the American Heart Association (AHA). One reason: high cholesterol. In fact, women tend to have higher cholesterol levels than men from age 45 on, according to the AHA. Flaxseed, which is rich in the omega-3 fat alpha-linoleic acid, may help lower it.

An Italian study of 40 male and female patients with cholesterol levels greater than 240 milligrams per deciliter found that consuming ground flaxseed (20 grams, or about 0.7 ounces, daily) could significantly lower levels of total and LDL cholesterol (the artery-clogging kind), while also improving the ratio of total cholesterol to HDL. (Low levels of HDL may be a greater risk factor for women, according to the AHA.) In a Harvard study of 76,763 women participating in the Nurses' Health Study, researchers also noted that women consuming a diet rich in alpha-linolenic acid seem to have a lower risk of dying from heart disease and stroke, compared with women whose diets were lacking this fat. Flaxseed also provides fiber; two tablespoons of ground flaxseed have 4 grams of fiber—almost 20% of the 25 grams recommended by the U.S. Department of Agriculture. Lignans, which are a particular type of fiber found in flaxseed, may also be beneficial for preventing breast and prostate cancer, according to preliminary studies. (Lignans are not present in flaxseed oil, however, notes integrative physician and herbalist Tieraona Low Dog, M.D.)

DOSAGE: Low Dog recommends adding 1 to 5 tablespoons of ground flaxseed to your diet several days a week; sprinkle it on cereal or yogurt, or stir it into protein shakes. Flaxseed oil—which must be kept refrigerated to prevent rancidity—should be added to salads and not used for cooking.

PRECAUTIONS: Flaxseed and its oil are safe if consumed in normal amounts, although they can produce a laxative effect. "If you eat huge amounts of flaxseed meal, you could develop cyanide toxicity, but this hasn't, to my knowledge, ever occurred in humans," says Low Dog.

7 GARLIC
(Allium sativum L.)

BEST FOR → **Ear infections and cancer prevention**

Garlic's antibiotic compound, alliin, has no medicinal value until the herb is chewed, chopped or crushed. Then an enzyme transforms alliin into a powerful antibiotic called allicin. Raw garlic has the most antibiotic potency, but garlic still has benefits when cooked. Garlic is antimicrobial and anti-inflammatory, so it will treat any infection, but when combined with mullein oil (*Verbascum densiflorum*), it's especially effective for ear infections, says a 2010 report in *Natural News*. The mullein oil is soothing, and helps draw out fluid to relieve pain and decrease pressure. According to the National Cancer Institute, preliminary studies in 2008 suggest that garlic consumption may also reduce the risk of developing several types of cancer, especially those of the gastrointestinal tract.

DOSAGE: Put three drops of oil in each affected ear, two to three times a day as needed. (The oils are sold in a premixed formula.) For internal use, fresh garlic or capsules may be used; follow label directions.

PRECAUTIONS: Don't put drops—or anything else—into your ear if you think the eardrum may be perforated.

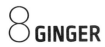

GINGER

(Zingiber officinale)

BEST FOR: Nausea and vomiting

A Danish study showed that new sailors prone to motion sickness had less vomiting than a placebo group. Research published in *Obstetrics & Gynecology* found that 88% of nausea-plagued pregnant women got relief when they took 1 gram a day of ginger powder for no longer than four days. And a 2008 study by *The Journal of Alternative and Complementary Medicine* found that powered ginger paired with high-protein meals eased chemotherapy-induced nausea.

DOSAGE: For motion sickness, take a 1-gram capsule of powdered gingerroot about an hour before you embark and another every two hours or as needed. For morning sickness, take 250 milligrams four times a day. Cooking with the herb may also be helpful.

PRECAUTIONS: Few side effects are linked to normal ginger consumption, but powdered ginger may produce bloating or indigestion. Ginger may also exacerbate heartburn in pregnant women.

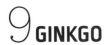

GINKGO

(Ginkgo biloba)

BEST FOR: Alzheimer's and antidepressant-induced sexual problems

In a landmark study published in *The Journal of the American Medical Association*, researchers gave 202 people with Alzheimer's either a placebo or 120 milligrams a day of ginkgo extract. A year later, the ginkgo group retained more mental function. According to new research in rats (2013), supplementation with an extract from *Ginkgo biloba* may help to battle memory loss and cognitive impairments associated with dementia by encouraging the growth and development of neural stem cells. From upstairs to downstairs: In a University of California, San Francisco study, investigators gave 209 milligrams of ginkgo a day to 63 people suffering from antide-pressant-induced sexual problems, including erection impairment, vaginal dryness and inability to reach orgasm; the herb helped 91% of the women and 76% of the men to return to normal sexual function.

DOSAGE: Traditional usage is 80 to 240 milligrams of a 50:1 standard-ized leaf extract daily or 30 to 40 milligrams of extract in a tea bag, prepared as a tea, for at least four to six weeks.

10 GINSENG

BEST FOR: Immune enhancement and diabetes

Many studies show that ginseng has "adaptogenic" powers, which means it helps the body adapt to stress and revs up the immune sys-tem. Most studies have used Panax *ginseng* (Asian ginseng). A 2013 University of Maryland review found that Asian ginseng may help boost the immune system, reduce risk of cancer and improve mental performance and wellbeing. And subjects who took daily doses of ginseng got fewer colds and less severe symptoms than a placebo group. Ginseng also reduces blood-sugar levels. A study in Toronto, Canada, found that Korean red ginseng improved glucose and insulin regulation in well-controlled type 2 diabetes. (Of course, diabetes requires professional treatment, so consult your physician about using ginseng.) Studies also have found ginseng supports liver func-tion and one preliminary study suggests that American ginseng (*Panax quinquefolius*), in combination with ginkgo (*Ginkgo biloba*), may help treat ADHD.

DOSAGE: 500 milligrams daily, best for short-term, stressful events

PRECAUTIONS: Should not be taken for more than six weeks. Avoid caffeine when taking ginseng, and do not take if pregnant.

11 GOLDENROD
(Solidago virgaurea)

BEST FOR: Nasal congestion

Goldenrod is particularly effective for treating congestion caused by allergies. Surprised? That's because goldenrod gets a bad rap. "People blame goldenrod for their allergies because they look across the field and see the beautiful yellow flowers," says herbalist Margi Flint, author of *The Practicing Herbalist.* "But it's the blooming ragweed they can't see that causes all the trouble. In nature, the remedy often grows right next to the cause." Also used for urinary infections and cystitis, and to flush out kidney and bladder stones.

DOSAGE: Place three drops of the extract under the tongue; repeat as necessary until nasal passages are clear.

12 GOLDENSEAL
(Hydrastis canadensis)

BEST FOR: Digestive-tract infections

Goldenseal, an herbal antibiotic, is often marketed in combination with echinacea as a treatment for infections, but it is effective only in the digestive tract, not for colds or flu. A 2012 University of Maryland study reported in *Clinical Advisor* found that goldenseal is an effective antibacterial agent and an aid to digestion. For gastrointestinal infections (e.g., ulcers, food poisoning, infectious diarrhea), ask your doctor about using goldenseal in addition to medical therapies. Also can be used topically for wounds and infections.

DOSAGE: For internal use, take a 300-milligram capsule three times a day; apply a dilution as needed for external use.

PRECAUTIONS: Can be toxic if taken to excess. May interact with antidepressants and codeine. Do not use if pregnant, nursing or suffering from high blood pressure.

13 LAVENDER
(Lavandula angustifolia)

BEST FOR: Headaches

"The scent of lavender triggers a calming response, releasing tension in the scalp muscles a bit, which eases the pain," explains Kingsbury Herbalist Rosemary Gladstar. She recommends using lavender oil in a pain-relieving foot soak: Add a few drops to a hot footbath, and then put a cold lavender-infused pack on the forehead. "This draws heat away from the head, and is guaranteed to make you feel better," she says.

DOSAGE: Dab a few drops of essential oil on each temple and rub some around the hairline. Breathe deeply and relax; repeat as needed.

PRECAUTIONS: Do not take the essential oil internally unless under the care of a professional.

14 LEMON BALM
(Melissa officinalis)

BEST FOR: Anxiety and herpes

Science has shown that lemon balm is tranquilizing. Several double-blind studies have found that a 600-milligram dose promoted calm and reduced anxiety. The herb and its oil have been used in Alzheimer's special care units to calm those who are agitated. To decompress after a tough day, try a cup of lemon balm tea; for extra benefit, mix with chamomile.

Lemon balm also has antiviral properties and has been shown to reduce the healing time of both oral and genital herpes. German researchers gave people in the early stages of herpes simplex virus outbreaks lemon balm cream or a placebo. The herb group had milder outbreaks that healed faster.

DOSAGE: Available in capsule form, tincture, and essential oil; follow label instructions.

PRECAUTIONS: Do not take the essential oil internally unless under the care of a professional.

15 MEADOWSWEET
(Filipendula ulmaria)

BEST FOR: Heartburn

The Native American herb, high in salicylic acid, calms inflammation in the stomach, often working within a day or two, says Sheila Kingsbury. "For people on protein pump inhibitors who are desperate to get their heartburn under control without medication, I have them drink one cup of meadowsweet tea a day, and that's all they need," she says. "They're always shocked that it's so easy."

DOSAGE: Pour 2 teaspoons of the dried herb in a cup of hot water; steep 20 minutes and drink once a day. (The slightly sweet tea has a mild almond flavor.)

PRECAUTIONS: Do not take meadowsweet if you're allergic to aspirin.

16 MILK THISTLE
(Silybum marianum)

BEST FOR: Liver health

Silymarin in milk thistle seeds has a remarkable ability to protect the liver. This herb has been shown to help treat hepatitis and alcoholic cirrhosis. "In our analysis," says Mark Blumenthal, executive director of the American Botanical Council, "a clear majority of studies support milk thistle seed extract for liver conditions." A 2010 NIH-NC-CAM study on the effects of silymarin on hepatitis C hepatology showed multiple positive effects demonstrating its antiviral and anti-inflammatory properties. Because most drugs are metabolized through the liver, many herbalists recommend silymarin for anyone who takes liver-taxing medication.

DOSAGE: 500 milligrams daily for liver health; also can be steeped in a tea.

17 PSYLLIUM
(Plantago spp.)

BEST FOR: **Digestive problems**

Psyllium is a tiny seed that contains mucilage, a soluble fiber that swells on exposure to water. For diarrhea, psyllium can absorb excess fluid in the gut. For constipation, psyllium adds bulk to stool, which presses on the colon wall and triggers the nerves that produce the urge to go. Also helps relieve hemorrhoids and helps remove toxins. May be used topically to draw out infections such as boils.

DOSAGE: Follow label directions; also available in capsule form.

PRECAUTIONS: When using psyllium, drink plenty of water; do not exceed recommended dose.

18 ST. JOHN'S WORT
(Hypericum perforatum)

BEST FOR: **Depression and pain**

"Long before it was ever used for depression or anxiety, St. John's wort was used as a pain reliever and an anti-inflammatory for muscle pains, burns, and bruises," explains Rosemary Gladstar, adding that blending the oil with the alcohol-based tincture helps draw the active constituents into the skin for faster healing. For mild depression, St. John's wort often works as well as some antidepressants but with fewer side effects. "We recently concluded a comprehensive review of the scientific literature on St. John's wort, and 21 of 23 studies support it for mild to moderate depression," says Blumenthal. It's not clear if

St. John's wort is as effective as selective serotonin reuptake inhibitors (SSRIs) such as Prozac or Zoloft, but a 2013 Mayo Clinic overview states that scientific evidence supports its use for mild to moderate depression; for severe depression, the evidence remains unclear.

DOSAGE: For depression, studies showing benefits have used 600 to 1,800 milligrams a day; most have used 900 milligrams a day. For pain, make a liniment by mixing equal parts St. John's wort tincture and St. John's wort oil. (Most concoctions come in 2-ounce bottles.) Mix vigorously before using, apply topically to affected area (avoiding the eyes), and massage into skin as needed.

PRECAUTIONS: Stomach upset is possible, and St. John's wort interacts with many drugs, including possibly reducing the effectiveness of birth control pills; so seek professional advice if you are taking a prescription medication. Depression requires professional care; ask your physician about St. John's wort. May cause sensitivity to light.

19 TEA TREE OIL
(Melaleuca alternifolia)

BEST FOR: Athlete's foot and other skin conditions

Tea tree is an Australian plant with an antifungal, antiseptic oil. In a double-blind trial, 158 people with athlete's foot were treated with a placebo, a 25% tea tree oil solution or a 50% tea tree oil solution for four weeks. Results showed that the tea tree oil solutions were more effective than placebo. (In the 50% tea tree oil group, 64% were cured; in the 25% tea tree oil group, 55% were cured; in the placebo group, 31% were cured.) Also helpful for a range of vaginal yeast infections.

DOSAGE: Apply essential oil mixed with a base cream or carrier oil to skin; for vaginal infections, use suppositories.

PRECAUTIONS: Do not take the essential oil internally unless advised by a professional.

20 TRIPHALA

(Emblica officinalis, Terminalia chebula and Terminalia belerica)

BEST FOR: Constipation and digestive problems

Triphala ("three fruits" in Sanskrit), a bowel-regulating formula in ayurvedic medicine, is a combination of the powdered fruits of amalaki, bibhitaki, and haritaki, all of which are rich sources of antioxidants with anti-inflammatory, adaptogenic, antistress, antibacterial, analgesic, anticancer and immune-enhancing properties. A 2012 review published in the *Chinese Journal of Integrative Traditional and Western Medicine* confirms the extensive healing properties of this amazing herbal compound.

"Triphala treats the entire digestive system, helping with constipation, hemorrhoids, diarrhea, indigestion, bloating and liver detoxification," explains ayurvedic herbalist Will Foster, L.Ac., who trained with traditional ayurvedic healers in India. Because it operates as a bowel tonic (helping to maintain proper function) rather than a laxative, triphala is safe to take every day.

DOSAGE: Take two to four 500-milligram tablets just before bedtime.

PRECAUTIONS: Do not take during pregnancy or if underweight; can cause weight loss.

21 TURMERIC

(Curcuma longa)

BEST FOR: Arthritis and cancer prevention

Curcumin, the active compound that gives the spice turmeric its bright-gold color, has long been known as an anti-inflammatory and antioxidant. In combination with boswellia, ashwagandha and ginger, it may treat osteoarthritis, according to a study published in the *Journal of Clinical Rheumatology.* And a recent study published in the journal *Phytotherapy* Research found curcumin to be "comparable" in efficacy to diclofenac sodium, a prescription anti-inflammatory, for treating rheumatoid arthritis.

The American Cancer Society has reported that large studies are being conducted to see how curcumin might prevent and treat cancer; one of the challenges is that it doesn't absorb well from the intestines, but that could be an advantage for targeting cancer precursors in the colon and rectum. For women with recurrent breast cancer, curcumin might prove especially useful; animal models have shown that curcumin may help prevent metastasis, even after failed treatment with the drug tamoxifen. In women with HER2-positive cancer, curcuminoids also seemed to behave much like the highly successful chemotherapy drug Herceptin, although research is very preliminary.

DOSAGE: It's best to get your curcumin by using turmeric in curries and other foods. If you aren't a fan of Indian food, take one 500-milligram capsule of curcumin—standardized to 95% curcuminoids—each day.

PRECAUTIONS: Side effects are rare but include flatulence, diarrhea and heartburn. Do not take turmeric if you're on blood thinners.

22 UMCKALOABO
(Pelargonium sidoides)

BEST FOR: Cough and cold

A really fun herb to pronounce, *umckaloabo* means "heavy cough" in Zulu. The South African herb is a powerhouse with antiviral and antibacterial properties, says herbalist Mark Blumenthal. "There are good clinical studies on the use of umckaloabo for treating bronchitis as well as tonsillitis," he says, adding that taking umckaloabo at the onset of symptoms will bring relief within a day or two. Recent

German studies of the preparation found that it significantly reduced symptoms and duration of colds and cough.

DOSAGE: Take as drops, syrups, chewable tablets or sprays. Follow package instructions.

23 WHITE WILLOW BARK
(Salix alba)

BEST FOR: Pain relief

White willow bark contains salicin, a close chemical relative of aspirin. A study in *Phytomedicine* followed people with severe back pain for 18 months. In the group taking white willow bark, 40% were pain-free after just four weeks; the same was true of only 18% of the second group, who were allowed to take whatever prescription drugs they wanted. In another well-designed study of nearly 200 people with low back pain, those who received willow bark experienced a significant improvement in pain compared to those who received placebo. People who received higher doses of willow bark (240 milligrams salicin) had more significant pain relief than those who received low doses (120 milligrams salicin). It has also been shown to relieve arthritis, inflammation, headaches and fever and hot flashes.

DOSAGE: Follow label directions; the bark can be made into a tea.

PRECAUTIONS: Like aspirin, willow bark can cause stomach distress, and shouldn't be given to children or used if pregnant or breast-feeding. Avoid if you are allergic to aspirin.

The Bliss Boosters

CHOCOLATE

Yes, chocolate is an herb, says "medicine hunter" Chris Kilham, ethnobotanist at the University of Massachusetts at Amherst. "Cocoa is one of the great herbal mood enhancers," he says. Chocolate contains a substance called anandamide—aka the bliss molecule—which is known to bind to human cannabinoid receptors (the same ones that interact with marijuana) to create a sense of well-being. "It's a bliss enhancer—*ananda* means bliss in Sanskrit," Kilham says. "We know that chocolate boosts natural levels of serotonin, the feel-good neurotransmitter. You can happily self-medicate with chocolate and greatly improve your brain chemistry."

STINGING NETTLE
(Urtica dioica)

Stinging nettle made its rep as an anti-allergy herb. But it's also a terrific energizer for women, says Susun Weed, master herbalist and author of the *Wise Woman Herbal* book series. "If you touch the wild stinging nettle plant, you will feel a shock—and that electricity and energy is available to us when we drink nettle infusion," says Weed. The benefits, she explains, are nearly endless:

Nettle restores and rebuilds the adrenal glands, tonifies the kidneys, rebuilds the pancreas and stabilizes blood sugar.

GOTU KOLA
(Centella asiatica)

It's hard to be happy when you can't think straight. According to Sheila Kingsbury, N.D., R.H., chairwoman of the Botanical Medicine Department at Bastyr University in Seattle, the solution for the inner muddle is gotu kola. "It's terrific for mood because it improves the flow of oxygen to the brain, making you feel awake and stimulated without feeling wired." (And this without a Diet Coke.)

MOTHERWORT
(Leonurus cardiaca)

When you're feeling anxious and want to run away and hide in that bag of Mint Milanos, try motherwort, a member of the mint family. "The Latin name means 'heart of the lion,'" says Weed.

   "That's exactly what motherwort does. It gives you the courage of the great cat. It's like sitting in your mother's lap."

MILKY OAT SEED
(Avena sativa)

Been burning the candle at both ends for so long your gut's on fire? This herb's for you, says David Winston, R.H., coauthor of the resource guide Winston and Kuhn's Herbal Therapy & Supplements.

Milky oat seed is—as the name implies—the extract of the whole milky oat produced by the oat plant in seed form only; you can't get similar benefits from, say, upping your morning oatmeal intake. "It creates a stronger and more balanced emotional foundation so that you're not as reactive to every little thing," Winston says. "It's an especially good choice for those people who make themselves sick with stress."

Flatten your belly—for good!

With
The 17-Day Green Tea Diet!

It seems incredible.
Impossible.
And yet it's true: Fast, permanent weight-loss
is just a sip away, thanks to this unique program
developed by the bestselling authors
of Eat This, Not That!

You'll get the:

★ **Complete, easy-to-use eating plan**

★ **Delicious recipes for meals, snacks, and even desserts**

★ **Day-by-day workout program to power fat burn**

You've tried the Cleanse—
now get results that last!

Buy
the e-book
today!

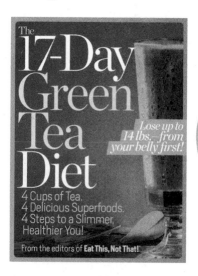

The companion
book for
*The 7-Day
Weight-Loss
Tea Cleanse!*

**AND FOR 1,000+ QUICK AND EASY WEIGHT-LOSS TIPS,
VISIT eatthis.com.**